'An intriguing series of self-portraits refracted through tender, sensitive meditations on art.'

– *Michèle Roberts*

'As a film maker, Jungian analyst, and writer, Juliet Miller has been continuously engaged with images, and aspects of the intense interface between life and art. The events she narrates in this sensitive memoir provide the reader with an opportunity to meditate on certain crucial moments in life when an encounter with a work of art can psychologically mirror, accompany, or challenge us, providing a temenos for self-analysis and healing. Her book will be of interest to therapists, art-lovers, and the general public.'

– *Diane Finiello Zervas is an art historian and Jungian analyst with the Independent Group of Analytical Psychologists*

'A compelling autobiography that teaches us the value of looking and listening to our inner reactions in our encounters with creative works. We readers move from exquisite descriptions of Juliet Miller's connections with paintings as a child, to seeing how her maturing life in art parallels and enhances her life as a psychoanalyst. She is a Jungian and as such the spiritual is never far away. What a pleasure to be alongside her developing understanding. This is a brilliant sequel to Juliet's previous books on art and creativity.'

– *Caroline Pick, film-maker and artist*

'Juliet Miller explores the nature, value and potential meaning(s) of art from within a Jungian depth psychology paradigm allied to a scholarly appreciation of art. Her understanding and use of this is central to the book and it is the emphasis on the experience of things, not theory (as Jung would value) that is the teacher here. We are encouraged to reflect more, stay still, listen closely and go deeper. Treasure to find and deep connections to make. Drawing together, and reflecting on different strands of her own rich experience, she helps us to think about art: the experience (and often difficult) processes of creation; engaging with it; and finding and making meaning. As a practising psychotherapist and artist I found this book illuminating and helpful.'

– *Sally Dhruev, psychotherapist and artist*

Art, Memoir and Jung

In this intimate study Juliet Miller maps the artworks that have influenced her throughout her life and examines how she has integrated them into her development as a psychotherapist.

Working from the premise that our initial reactions to art provide a crucial key to self-analysis, Miller interrogates the significance of different artists, including Bourgeois, Vermeer, Rousseau and Kahlo, and analyzes how personal circumstances, recollections and emotions have affected responses to their work. Chapters incorporate clinical material from Miller's practice, linking into her own anxieties about sitting with and connecting with patients, and touching on themes including creativity, character, identity and communication.

Through this exploration she questions many of the conventions of art and psychotherapy and suggests ways in which looking at art can be used as a psychological tool. *Art, Memoir and Jung* offers a highly personal and innovative perspective on meaning in art and how it can be used to explore Jungian thought as based in the aesthetic, and how the aesthetic can inform depth psychology.

Juliet Miller is a writer and Jungian analyst based in the UK. She is fascinated by the interface between art and psyche. She is also the author of *The Creative Feminine and her Discontents: Psychotherapy, Art and Destruction*.

Art, Memoir and Jung

Personal and Psychological Encounters

Juliet Miller

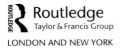

LONDON AND NEW YORK

First published 2021
by Routledge
2 Park Square, Milton Park, Abingdon, Oxon OX14 4RN

and by Routledge
52 Vanderbilt Avenue, New York, NY 10017

Routledge is an imprint of the Taylor & Francis Group, an informa business

© 2021 Juliet Miller

The right of Juliet Miller to be identified as author of this work has been asserted by her in accordance with sections 77 and 78 of the Copyright, Designs and Patents Act 1988.

All rights reserved. No part of this book may be reprinted or reproduced or utilized in any form or by any electronic, mechanical, or other means, now known or hereafter invented, including photocopying and recording, or in any information storage or retrieval system, without permission in writing from the publishers.

Trademark notice: Product or corporate names may be trademarks or registered trademarks, and are used only for identification and explanation without intent to infringe.

British Library Cataloguing-in-Publication Data
A catalogue record for this book is available from the British Library

Library of Congress Cataloging-in-Publication Data
Names: Miller, Juliet, 1946- author.
Title: Art, memoir and Jung : personal and psychological encounters / Juliet Miller.
Description: 1 Edition. | New York : Routledge, 2020. | Includes bibliographical references and index. |
Identifiers: LCCN 2020020713 (print) | LCCN 2020020714 (ebook) | ISBN 9780367537173 (hardback) | ISBN 9780367537180 (paperback) | ISBN 9781003083030 (ebook)
Subjects: LCSH: Jungian psychology. | Psychotherapy. | Psychology and art.
Classification: LCC BF173.J85 M55 2020 (print) | LCC BF173.J85 (ebook) | DDC 150.19/54–dc23
LC record available at https://lccn.loc.gov/2020020713
LC ebook record available at https://lccn.loc.gov/2020020714

ISBN: 978-0-367-53717-3 (hbk)
ISBN: 978-0-367-53718-0 (pbk)
ISBN: 978-1-003-08303-0 (ebk)

Typeset in Times
by River Editorial Ltd, Devon, UK

For Amelia and Verity

Contents

	Acknowledgements	xi
1	Shock	1
2	Affected by art	5
3	The gaze	14
4	Red paint	22
5	Stillness	31
6	Touch	39
7	Beads and threads	47
8	Struggle	55
9	Multiple selves	64
10	Space	71
11	The dream	79
12	Silence	88
13	Alchemy	96
14	The heretic	107

15	Walking	116
16	Afterword	125
	Bibliography	128
	Index	131

Acknowledgements

Thanks are due to the following people:

For their consistent support for this book, my writing colleagues Thea Abbott and Adrian Ward who have stuck with me and it for five years.
To Caroline Pick for generously sharing her acute visual sense.
To Penelope Cherns for her boundless creative energy.
To Barbara Derkow for her constant support.
To Mimi Potworowska for showing me how artistic endeavour is directly related to psychotherapy.
To my agent Jessica Woolard.
Thanks are also due to my patients and supervisees who have kept reminding me why art is important.
As always my special thanks are due to David Arnold whose steady presence I could not do without.

I am especially grateful to the following art institutions and copyright holders:

Bridgeman Images
National Gallery, London
Musées Royaux des Beaux-Arts de Belgique, Belgium
Dublin City Art Gallery, The Hugh Lane Bequest, Ireland
The Courtauld Gallery, London
Mrs Simon Guggenheim Fund, The Museum of Modern Art, New York
Scala Archives
Chapel of the Cemetery, Monterchi, Italy, Bridgeman Images
Raffaello Bencini
Kettle's Yard, University of Cambridge
Christie's Images
Art Gallery of Ontario
De Agostini Picture Library
M. Steemuller
Banco de Mexico Diego Rivera Frida Kahlo Museum Trust
Museum of Modern Art, Mexico

DACS
Museo di San Marco, Florence
Musée d'Orsay, Paris
Luisa Ricciarini
Gemaeldegalerie Alte Meister, Dresden
Staatliche Kunstsammlungen, Dresden
The Estate of Howard Hodgkin
The Easton Foundation
Allan Finkelman
Glenstone Foundation
Christopher Burk
Richard Long
New Art Centre, Roche Court Sculpture Park
Houghton Hall, Norfolk

Chapter 1

Shock

During a damp Saturday morning in February many years ago, my phone rang. I was contemplating the delights of the weekend ahead – there was a film to look forward to and later on supper with friends. I quickly registered that it was my sister on the phone but I couldn't understand her jumbled words, it was as if they were in a strange foreign language. When she had repeated herself a few times I was finally able to take in what she was saying, 'Dad has died. Dad has died'.

'What do you mean? How do you know?' My disbelief was intense. My father had been fit and well when I last saw him and he was enjoying making a new garden in Oxfordshire. There had been no suggestion that he was ill. My sister was staying with our parents and when he had not responded to her call for 'coffee!' she had gone outside and found him lying beside the newly dug earth of a rose bed. He was already cold to her touch.

I was enjoying a busy new life of my own in London and was completely unprepared for this explosion of death into our family. I spent the following week with my mother and two siblings arranging the funeral, and trying to take in what had happened. It made no sense to me at all. How could someone whom I loved dearly simply leave like that? I was close to my father. We didn't do much together or have long conversations, but we seemed to understand each other's moods and ways of seeing the world. But now I was acutely aware of all the many conversations with him I had not had and which I would now never have. I'd been waiting to have these delayed delights when I was less absorbed in my own interests and needs, imagining always that there would be plenty of time ahead. Now that fantasy future had vanished and he'd gone without so much as a 'goodbye'.

In that unreal time that has to be got through between a death and a funeral, my grief seemed to be primarily physical and I felt very unwell. My heart pounded irregularly in my chest, I slept briefly and deeply as if I had been drugged and then I would wake with a start to find myself alive somehow, but suffocated with grief. I shut myself in the loo and howled, surprising myself with the animal noises I was making. We clustered together as a family trying to support each other, yet I soon realized that

2 Shock

the experience of grief is such an individual affair that it is difficult to share with anyone, most of all family. For each of us he was an individual and unique father or husband. Loyalties and sibling rivalries were recalled, forcing their uncomfortable presence into the mourning space – who had loved most, who had been loved most, who had understood him the most? We had all loved in such different ways and needed to grieve these differences alone. Sometimes I took myself off to my father's study and closed the door. I tried sniffing his chair and his books to see whether I could recall his unique and comforting body odour. I persuaded myself that if I concentrated hard enough on his presence the door would open and he would walk in. My ability to accept what had happened lagged way behind what appeared to be the reality. My shocked brain was taking its time to compute.

It is I suppose some consolation when someone dies prematurely that their funeral is well attended. At my father's funeral there were lots of saddened friends and family. Afterwards their flowers lay in a long row down a hard concrete path in the crematorium. There were wreaths and bunches of flowers, some small intimate posies with heart-rending personal messages on them and also some grand bouquets. I couldn't bear that all these flowers would be left on this cold concrete slab, where no one who knew my father would see them, and so I requested that they were brought back to the house. There, for a few hours in a fugue-like state, I unwound flowers from wreaths, placed them in water and rescued pierced stems from sharp, binding wire, willing I suppose for some kind of resurrection.

A couple of days later I returned to London. I had taken a couple of weeks off work and now had a grey empty void stretching in front of me. I had no idea what to do. I found myself taking long hot baths in the middle of the day, waiting for my body to show some signs of life, or was it the opposite, hoping for a form of self-immolation? I couldn't believe that there was any future in which I would have a part, or that the world could continue to exist without my father in it. Then, about a week after the funeral, I dreamt that he was sitting in my sitting room opposite me and smiling. That I could bring his physical form to life in this way encouraged me that I had not lost him entirely.

After a few days I forced myself to go out into the bleak February weather and went into town. I hadn't thought much about where I would go but found myself in Trafalgar Square. I was feeling skinless and vulnerable and welcomed the sight of the National Gallery as a refuge. Here it was quiet and warm. I was incapable of taking in any of the paintings, but felt reassured by their ongoing silent presence. Out of habit I had gravitated toward the rooms housing the Impressionists and I sat down on a bench in front of a painting by Degas of a portrait of a young woman, *Helen Rouart in her Father's Study* (Figure 1.1).

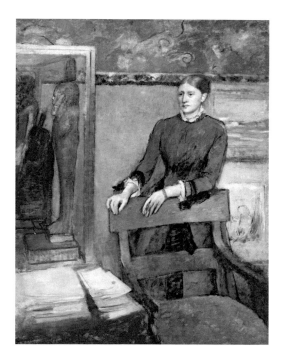

Figure 1.1 Helen Rouart in her Father's Study, Edgar Degas, oil on canvas, 1886.
© National Gallery, London, UK/Bridgeman Images.

After a while I realized that my shattered concentration had come together enough for me to begin to look at it. It is a large reddish-brown painting. Helen is standing behind her father's oversized empty chair, with her arms resting on it. She is an elegant figure with her red hair drawn back and she is wearing a fitted grey dress with a small lace collar. She is looking out of the picture but her eyes are slightly glazed as if her concentration is elsewhere. She is contemplating her own thoughts whilst expecting her father to return. Papers are piled on the desk next to the chair and in a glass case behind this are some Egyptian funereal wooden figures. This is a man's private working space, which reflects his own internal world, and in which his daughter is waiting for him, or maybe for some revelation of her own. It is a painting about absence.

As I kept looking at this attentive and waiting daughter I felt a small shift in the leadenness of my grief, as if a chink had opened up to allow space for a different feeling. The relief was immense as, for probably only a couple of seconds, I had understood that my desolation would not kill me because I had been noticed by this painting. It was as if I had experienced a tiny electric charge registering on an internal meter, that I was not completely dead to the world. Degas had seen inside me, and shown my feelings to me in paint. There was a similarity between Helen's quiet expectancy in her father's study and my own desolate longings. My grief had made me very lonely, but whilst looking at this painting I felt met and understood by paint on canvas. I had seen and admired the painting before, but this time it was in tune with my state of mind and I felt it was there entirely for me. After a while I went to the shop and bought a postcard of *Helen Rouart in her Father's Study*. For a long time I kept it in my bag, as if it was a photo of someone I loved and whom I wanted to keep close. It was a constant reminder, as I slowly became used to my father's absence, that art had the capacity to lead me back to myself, touch places in me that otherwise seemed inaccessible and remind me who I was.

Art has continued to inform my life in this reflective way. Sometimes it has met me where I am, and sometimes it has moved me on. It has shaken me up, irritated, annoyed, placated and soothed me. It has wrapped me in warmth or given my life meaning when there seemed to be none. Most importantly, it has asked questions of me and required me to respond. It has been a most demanding and persistent companion and one that has forced me to look at what it is that binds us so closely together, on both a conscious and unconscious level. Sometimes it has been a mirror and sometimes a questioning friend. I now think of my relationship with art as intense, and life-long and as a form of self-analysis which has made me wonder about the origins of this partnership and to question how it all began, a long time before I became a Jungian analyst myself.

Chapter 2

Affected by art

I was aware that paintings could engender powerful responses in me when I was quite young. I was a shy introverted child with two siblings but few friends and we grew up in a large, draughty and rather bleak house which my parents had bought after the war; not bomb damaged exactly, but a suffering structure with leaks and draughts, unattended to after London's exhausting ordeal. The house was permanently freezing, the temperature completely unaffected by one-bar electric fires, and I was always miserably cold. On the top landing there was a large metal bowl, just outside my bedroom door, which caught insistent and infuriating sleep-denying drips from the leaking roof. A lot of the wallpaper was peeling or had been picked at and torn along the joins by small, intrusive hands. The floorboards were painted black to hide the gaps where the rugs didn't meet and the windows rattled and creaked in their ill-fitting frames, but I loved the dilapidated house. The windows were large and looked out onto a sometimes green, sometimes dusty London square, and on sunny days mote-filled beams of light bent themselves through the waves in the Georgian glass and rushed across the rooms.

Because of my love for the house and also my need for security, I had a recurrent anxious dream that it became unstable, reflecting maybe early anxieties about my own psychological strengths. The tall structure would shudder and the stairs would threaten to collapse, but on waking I was always reassured by my parents that it would stay upright despite needing lots of attention. There was no money for repairs and so my parents, in an attempt not to worry, tried to forget about them. Anyway there was something far more important to be preoccupied with than a new roof or heating, something that the family could not apparently do without, and that was paintings. Considering that my mother was trained as an architect this privileging of art over the substance of a house was considered odd by some of her friends, but entirely normal by us children. I felt safer when reading books than meeting people, but my family's belief in a parallel world of art gave me an identity to hang on to in social situations. It didn't seem to increase my standing among my school friends, or help me to be understood by them, but loving paintings was the closest my family could get to embracing an organized religion, and as a result it felt like we belonged to something.

Belonging meant that I would be given precious talismans from galleries. A postcard of *Tiger in a Tropical Storm (Surprised!)* by Rousseau would be propped against a bowl of potatoes during supper, making me long to see this exotic wet tiger for myself. *La Loge* by Renoir would be attached to a book for my birthday with a promise of tickets for the ballet, or Van Gogh's *Bedroom at Arles* would carry a message on the back from my father when he was away, saying 'sleep well'.

My parents had met late in the war, married within two months and were then separated for two and a half years when my father was sent to Russia to work on an allied Russian/British newspaper. The rushed war marriage had its roots in shared political views, a love of reading and a highly individual visual sense. It was this mutual love of painting and sculpture that helped to re-cement the post-war marriage when my parents had to get to know each other again and bring up a family. My brother, sister and I grew up with these signs of commitment displayed all over the house, and since childhood I have always felt that life without books and especially pictures would be terrifyingly empty and relationship-less. I think that I was probably dimly aware that although paintings were 'things', they were not quite like other things, and that loving a painting was somehow different from loving my father's armchair or the curtains in my room.

Art was part of our daily language, and the everyday world was frequently referred to in painterly terms; *that plate is Picasso-esque or that field looks just like a Corot*. It was as if it was painters who understood the real nature of things and how they fitted into and reflected the feelings and emotions of the world. I was aware that there might be some snobbery inherent in these comments, as certain artists would be dismissed as not coming within the charmed circle of those who could see in this way. But my parents' tastes were relatively broad and ranged from the Italian Renaissance to modern artists of their time such as Braque and Giacometti. The walls were covered with reproductions of all the Van Goghs, Degas, Monets and Picassos that could be squeezed in. In amongst this cornucopia of masterpieces some original paintings and prints were also given wall space – the paintings of a great uncle, Claude Flight, who had developed the lino-cut tradition, the oil painting of a white horse in a dark forest by an admirer of my mother, my mother's own competent watercolours, my father's Russian posters and my sister's and my attempts to emulate any favoured artist of the moment. Each piece of paper or framed picture, whether an original or a reproduction, had its own recognized position in the house and its own unique relationship with the members of the family.

Mr and Mrs Andrews by Gainsborough (Figure 2.1) greeted us sternly when we entered the hall. The aristocratic couple looked out at our damp London house from their privileged position on their grand country estate. Mr Andrews, resplendent in his silk jacket, velour britches and three-cornered hat, was the master of all he surveyed; the gun, the dog, the wife in her blue satin dress and the landscape as far as the eye could see. I interpreted the slight smirk on Mr Andrews' face as a response to the dilapidated state of our hall and also as a constant reminder that although we were now separated by two centuries, the English upper classes remained defiantly in charge. I was fascinated by the imbalance in the painting with the couple posing on the left-hand side and the great open space of their valuable land on the right-hand side. This unpopulated vista of fields and trees drew me into an exclusive world of wealth and privilege.

I had been told about the context of the painting and that Gainsborough had been required to paint a portrait of the couple, but also, significantly, that he had to show their position and wealth and to reflect their own sense of importance. This was a painting to help shore up the couple against any threat of change. They had enough money and status to believe that the world that Gainsborough was reflecting for them would remain exactly the same. The awkwardness and rigidity of the figures didn't disturb me then, and I looked at the painting every day in the kind of unfocussed way one looks at familiar objects, as long as they remain in

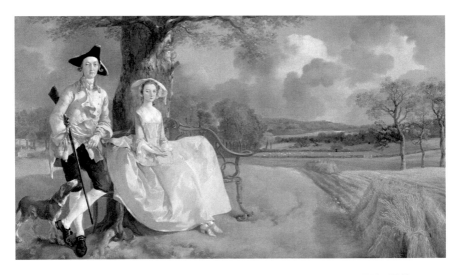

Figure 2.1 Mr and Mrs Andrews, Thomas Gainsborough, oil on canvas, c.1748–1749.
© National Gallery London, UK/Bridgeman Images.

the right place. It was a solace and comfort for me too, a reassurance that all remained the same in my world also. *Mr and Mrs Andrews* was a familiar of this kind, a protection against external threat. The painting belonged to us, as it lived permanently in the hall, so much so that when I happened to see the original in the National Gallery I was momentarily shocked that it had been removed from its rightful home.

Mr and Mrs Andrews had not always lived with us. We had given the print to our parents on their wedding anniversary in appreciation of the artist but also as an ironic comment, or so my siblings and I thought, on their own marriage, which was neither subordinate nor wealthy. So the reproduction only appeared in the house when I was a teenager, and maybe because of their sense of entitlement the couple were given pride of place in the hall, thereby sending a small and unobtrusive Monet print, which no one seemed to care much about, scuttling off to the basement to live in isolation with the lodger. Although prominent in the hall the Andrews' domain went no further. Although they exuded continuity and reliability, they lacked imagination and with their coolness and acceptance of their superior position I felt it would have been dangerous to allow them closer to the sitting room or even upstairs where the house was warmer and the paintings more exuberant. The couple, because they were a late addition to an eclectic collection of pictures, were never quite taken into our hearts. They were kept firmly in the draughty hall away from the main rooms and were therefore allowed to exert less power than the group of long established and entrenched occupants.

The picture that dominated the sitting room was an enormous print of Van Gogh's *Sunflowers*. The viridian green background was a startling contrast to the thick yellow and black of the dropping flower heads. I was intrigued by the way Van Gogh had signed his name in an arc around the vase, rather than in a corner at the bottom of the canvas, almost as if he was naming the flowers as himself, a form of self-portrait. I still feel the same as I did then about his paintings, as if they are thick, brilliant explosions of soul. The sunflowers were well on their way to becoming seed heads and simultaneously oozed energy and decay, hope and sadness. The painting conveyed an urgent message of transience that was both exhilarating and despairing and so completely unlike the rigid frozen world of the Gainsborough. Van Gogh had painted it in 1888 to hang in the room he was preparing for Gauguin, whom he was hoping was going to stay with him in the Yellow House in Arles that 'shone out' from the surroundings (Gayford, 2007: 14). It was one of six paintings Van Gogh had hung in the room his friend was to stay in. Our reproduction brought into our sitting room some of the artist's intense desire to be understood and loved by his friend. Without understanding the dynamics of this doomed friendship, I responded to Van Gogh's desire with my own devotion – a devotion to the way in which the large brush marks had twisted the paint onto the canvas, splaying open the hairs of the brush head in feathered arcs, to the contrasts and surprising clashes of yellow, black and blue/green paint and most of all to the energy and wildness of it all.

I was always under the impression that our reproduction was larger than the actual canvas, maybe because of its dominant position above the sofa, or maybe simply because the painting commanded so much of my attention. I was surprised to discover later that it was in fact the same size as the original. Our reproduction must have been a good one, as the thick layers of paint appeared to be three dimensional behind the glass. In the twenty years my parents had the house, the *Sunflowers* in all its exuberant display of painterly ability was never dislodged from its commanding position.

In the back of the sitting room where we ate, there was a small hatch in the wall through which plates could be passed to the kitchen. Beside this there was just enough wall room for *Landscape with the Fall of Icarus* by Bruegel (Figure 2.2). I grew up thinking that there was only one version of this painting. In ours, Icarus had already fallen into the sea and all you could see of him was his leg sticking up at a strange angle out of the water.

Nowadays this version is considered to be a copy and in the original a wax-winged Icarus is still flying close to the sun testing his wings. The true Bruegel however still feels like that reproduction hanging next to

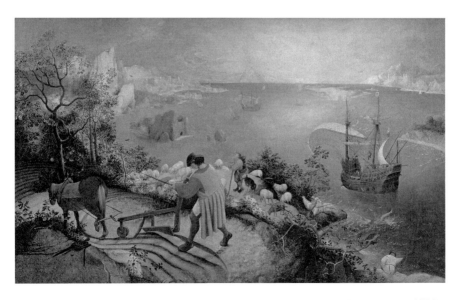

Figure 2.2 Landscape with the Fall of Icarus, Pieter Bruegel the Elder, oil on canvas, c.1558. © Musées Royaux des Beaux-Arts de Belgique, Belgium/Bridgeman Images.

the kitchen hatch. Every day over breakfast I would stare at Icarus' bent leg sticking out of the sea and the ploughman in his strange skirt. I was a slow riser and I hated breakfast. It was always too early, too rushed and too indigestible. It was much easier to look at the painting rather than face my congealing egg. *Landscape with the Fall of Icarus* reassured me that time could indeed be frozen. In the painting there is no pressure to eat, or rush to catch the bus to school. Despite impending disaster the world continues to turn and to go about its business, all remains the same. Icarus' leg would be in the same position when I got home. With the uncertainties of the school day looming I found this very consoling.

To this day I could draw the entire structure of this painting from memory. My daily scanning of every inch of reproduced canvas over breakfast added to my sense of the brilliance and importance of the work and also to the strange feeling that my knowledge of the work was reciprocated. I felt that the picture knew me too and had found a way to get inside me; that my close examination of this framed piece of cardboard involved a two-way process and that the shapes made by the curving furrows on the ploughed field would never leave me, as if they had in some way etched themselves onto my retina forever. The dropping folds of the ploughman's smock, the rounded back of his thick hair and the worrying right-angle made by Icarus' bare leg sticking out of the sea appeared sometimes in one of my dreams and then became animated, as if to express they were looking for a permanent place where they could fit inside me and reside.

In my parents' bedroom there was a pale green and pink vase of flowers by Odilon Redon, ethereal and subtle and easy to love, and then two reproductions of black-ink drawings from Picasso's *Vollard Suite* involving a minotaur and naked women, which made my prepubescent self anxious. I wasn't sure I liked the idea of a minotaur and naked women in close proximity to each other, and the artist's confidence with line made me uneasy. It seemed all too easily done and as a result I wasn't sure how much Picasso cared about what his prodigious talent produced. A residue of that concern has affected my attitude towards the artist ever since. Maybe my fantasies about my parents' bedroom, which consisted of midnight longings to creep into their bed, as well as fearing the room a bit as it was frequently out of bounds, was more to do with these early reactions to Picasso than it was to any Oedipal longings.

My sister's chosen reproductions were the speckled delights of Bonnard and Vuillard, interiors full of light and flowers and bruised colours. My brother's tiny bedroom walls were covered in reproductions of early Italian painters, an especial hero being Piero della Francesca. My room was home to any Renoir reproduction that I could find, and later to any Matisse.

Although we did have a few paintings that had been done by friends and relatives, it was the reproductions of famous works that sought and got the family's attention. These reproductions were treated almost as if they were originals and they were framed as such. The *Sunflowers* had a bevelled frame painted in gold. *Mr and Mrs Andrews* had a delicate thin white frame with an inlay of brown stain and *Landscape with Icarus* had a plain oak frame that had housed many other reproductions before it. These cast off old loves had been left in the frame to provide a bit of padding behind the paper-thin work of Pieter Bruegel the Elder, which now rippled with damp behind the glass. In the days before cheap clip frames our fragile paper art treasures were presented with dignity and reverence, and I grew up believing that the pictures my parents chose for the house had a potent aura about them; similar to icons, they drew us into a world of paint and reverence. They were *our* pictures and they seemed to have acquired the power to know us as much as we knew them. They affected us but were also affected by us and were imbued with the characteristics of the walls and rooms of the house we lived in. Like old family pets they smelled of us and bore the scars of living with us. They became so familiar that they dropped off our conscious radar having found a permanent home in our internal visual vocabularies.

Over time I appear to have assimilated specific works of art as if they were an innate part of me. I do not mean that I believed that I could paint or draw like the artist, but rather that the works spoke to me so intensely and were received in such a similar vein that they became an indelible part of my experiencing of the world.

My mother had a very determined approach to her domestic environment, moulding the house as much as she could to her artistic ends with no money. Colour and instant results were far more important than preparation or precision. Her erratic decorating habits sometimes resulted in splashes of paint appearing on the frames and glass as she worked around the pictures rather than removing them from the walls. With the critical eye of a child I used to think that this was entirely due to laziness. I now wonder whether she was loath to disturb the pictures from their designated homes because she was wary of the power they held. Sometimes reproductions were allowed to remain, despite fading dramatically where the evening sun had caught them. *Ville Industrielle*, an early Van Gogh landscape of factories and smoke, had lost some of its original vigour on the left-hand side, where the sun crept round a curtain edge, but it was loved despite this diminishment. *The Sunflowers* hung for years glassless but resplendent in its gold frame after the glass smashed when the reproduction fell off the wall of its own accord in the middle of one night.

After my siblings and I had left home and my parents finally moved house, some of these beloved reproductions were hung in a series of bedsits and flats where they held a talismanic ability to transform any small damp space into a feasible place to live. I still have the gold frame from the *Sunflowers* although the reproduction faded into a pale green and brown blur years ago, as if the image had been so thoroughly absorbed into the family that it was no longer needed as an external object, for it had entered us all and now lived inside us.

Being excited by paintings outshone any experience I had at school. When I was eight, my sister and I started travelling on the tube together to the French Lycee. My parents had made this uncharacteristic and rather strange decision to take us out of the English school system with the sole purpose of getting us to speak French. They were right about us learning French, but maybe unaware of the rigid French educational system, which favours equality over independence and creativity, and I felt lost and isolated. The journey was an ordeal of crowded smoke-filled tube carriages and anxiety about our safety and being late. The school days then dragged and I resigned myself to surviving them, picking up my sister and getting back home as fast as possible. Most of my school hours were spent in the grip of a profound boredom, and a sense that any initiative on my part was not welcomed. At home I could read what I wanted and make my own paintings. Our house with its lack of physical comforts and its eccentricities was where experimentation could happen. From school I would bring back small cramped drawings on tiny bits of regulated school paper, which my mother looked at with distain and I was then ashamed of and threw away.

At home there was always plenty of paper – the back of my father's rejected foolscap typed sheets or, much better, rolls of lining paper which could be spread out on the floor and pinned down by books at the corners. These tempting cream expanses could be painted on with abandon with large brushes and thick poster paints, far superior to the thin, insipid powder paints supplied at school. Dragging colours across the paper or blobbing them on top of each other and trying to avoid the inevitable muddy purple-brown that resulted, seemed to me infinitely more purposeful than the constricted drawings that I did at school. As I dipped my brush into a pot of gleaming yellow paint I'd feel my anxious self slip away and I'd enter a new territory where I allowed myself fantasies of making brush marks like the ones in Van Gogh's *Sunflowers*, willing my lining paper to become canvas and my paint to take on the lusciousness of oil.

I sent one of my painting attempts, which I called *Blossoming Fruit Trees*, into a children's painting competition and was stunned to receive a paint box as a prize, only then to be told that there had been a mistake and that I hadn't won third prize. My mother insisted that I send the already used paint box back, despite the humiliation this entailed. A week later a letter arrived saying I had won the first prize and a bicycle instead. This was considered such an unlikely event that when I read the letter to my parents they didn't believe me. The bicycle duly arrived however and was a welcome tool of independence and a constant reminder of the power of paint.

My appetite for paint was encouraged by the bicycle but more powerfully by my first visits to art galleries. However much I may have revered our reproductions it was as nothing compared with the feelings aroused when looking at the actual art works. In a gallery I could stand in front of a Van Gogh and know that the artist had made this mark, the mark that I had admired in reproduction, by pressing his thick brush into the canvas, this canvas. I could see the amount of pressure he had exerted and the little twist he had given the brush as he removed it again. I could appreciate the amount of oil he had added by the way the undulating surface shimmered as if it had been painted yesterday. It was as if I was standing next to the artist himself.

In front of a painting by Corot I could almost hear the intake of breath as the painter dabbed his pointed brush in cadmium red and then, with a delicate touch, gave his small figure in the landscape a tiny but crucial triangle of a hat. In front of a Renoir painting I could see the true nature of that remarkable blue paint which was never entirely replicated by any of the other Impressionists. These were the real things, made by the artists' hands and they were full of snippets of seductive information that were not there to be appreciated in any reproduction, however good.

The first works that I saw in galleries physically enmeshed me in ways that took my breath away. I was overwhelmed by the intensity of my responses to real paint on canvas and fascinated by the visceral ways my body responded. As James Elkins the art historian writes: 'Paint incites motions, or the thought of motions, and through them it implies emotions and other wordless experiences' (Elkins, 1999: 193). It appeared that looking at paintings might not just involve my eyes but might engage my body with responses as well.

Chapter 3

The gaze

Renoir, the voluptuous, blowsy painter of female flesh and elegant women is not considered an interesting artist by many contemporary critics and is now rather out of fashion. When I was growing up my parents thought of Renoir as too pretty and probably a bit vulgar and therefore rather insubstantial as a painter; Pissarro, Van Gogh and Gauguin were preferred. When I was taken to the National Gallery aged ten, immune to my parents' preferences, I fell in love immediately with Renoir's *Les Parapluies* and claimed it for myself (Figure 3.1). This painting introduced me to the world of thick, viscous, glorious paint. Falling in love with Renoir also encouraged in me an awareness of my physical self, both as seen by others and self-experienced. When I think of Renoir now, I do so with a fondness for the painter who first showed me what paint could do, how to look at it and how to be aware of myself looking at it.

Les Parapluies was in some ways a classic painting for a ten-year-old girl to fall in love with. It features two young girls amidst a crowd of adults with their umbrellas up, and it is a pretty picture in an obvious way, although it was far more than this initial prettiness that excited me. It was as if I had stepped through a blue Renoir filter into a place where the external world was less delineated than I had experienced it before. The painter was showing me how he saw things and I realised that I could see them like that too. This was highlighted by my feeling that no one else could ever have felt as intensely about this painting as I did. This fantasy was probably helped by the fact that at that time no one else in my family *was* interested in Renoir, so he belonged to me and I could enjoy my righteous appreciation.

I can remember the sense of being overwhelmed with blue and being drawn to the foreground figures of the two girls who were on my level and directly in my eye line. I identified with the taller of the two; she had red hair like mine, emerging from her bonnet. The smaller girl, holding her hoop and looking directly at me, reminded me of my younger sister. What could be more enticing than discovering that we were inside a painting that hung in the National Gallery? Although I was a tubby and rather messy child I harboured ideas of metamorphosing into something rather different.

The gaze   15

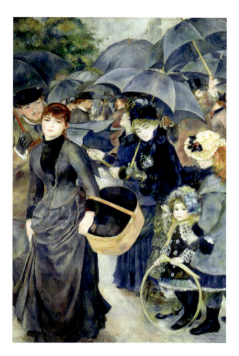

Figure 3.1 Les Parapluies, Pierre-Auguste Renoir, oil on canvas, 1886.
© Dublin City Art Gallery, The Hugh Lane Bequest, Ireland, Bridgeman Images.

How wonderful it would be to wear little black boots and bonnets and velvet-edged coats with lace collars! I think that I was aware of the young woman on the left of the picture who has a basket over her arm and is pulling her skirt up out of the wet, as someone whom I might become. A man seems to be speaking to her, maybe accosting her from over her shoulder. but she pays no notice and looks straight out of the picture directing her gaze back at the viewer; she, like the youngest girl on the right, is looking at us, or as I fantasised, just at me. I existed for both the woman and the girl as a gazing or even a staring stranger.

The sense of being noticed had a potent effect on me as a child. My shyness made me feel invisible and I was used to watching others rather than being watched myself. This was probably a trait that was helpful in me becoming a psychotherapist later in life, but at that early stage it felt like a major disadvantage. So when I first saw *Les Parapluies* it was exhilarating to feel that the picture was looking at me and I fantasised that the painter knew I was there. This seemed to be a more benign form of being noticed, with none of the attendant concerns about how I might be seen by another person in the street or at school. I appeared to be OK just as I was.

I felt that I could catch the ripples of blue light emanating from the canvas and I persuaded myself that no one else felt them or even knew that they were there. A sense of specialness seemed to be crucial to this baptism. Drowning in blue paint I had a first glimpse of what lay beneath the surface, a chance to make a connection with the mind of an artist. Renoir seemed to be inviting me into the picture and as a result I felt that my gaze mattered to him. This thought brought with it a thrill as I became aware that looking at pictures could be a two-way process and not just be about me passively looking. It seemed that it involved a very active engagement on an emotional level. The painter and I could, between us, create new undiscovered worlds. This was very exciting and the sense of intimacy it offered was novel. Just like I would eventually discover through an early love affair, I had little concept of what lay beneath, except a fascination for whatever might be there.

This awareness of desire was a new, intense and somewhat illicit kind of relationship involving exciting feelings not encountered before. I felt that my relationship with the artist was private, a secret affair, although my family teased me openly about my adoration. I experienced Renoir's use of paint and brushstrokes as a highly sensuous experience; the way he stippled the paint to form texture on clothes and hats and then followed the female forms in their delicious and luxuriant clothes with smooth blue strokes. The artist was showing himself to me in an attempt to discover whether I felt likewise. I could admire and love his work and be important to him in the process, which fed my own desire for admiration. He seemed to be saying *this is who I am. Do you like me?* There was also a sense of unknown depths, as if the painting was unconsciously holding the tensions of my pre-pubertal years under a surface of quiet respectable blueness. As Elkins suggests: 'We want to *be* pictures, not just be in them' (Elkins, 1996: 85).

After that first encounter with *Les Parapluies* I remember leaving the gallery with my father and coming out into Trafalgar Square, which now seemed broken up into patches of colour. The boundaries between buildings and backgrounds had become blurred and the fountains and the grey pavement were far bluer than I had remembered them an hour before. Rain the colour of bluebells was falling over the Square. Everything looked like a Renoir. The painter had got into me and infected my way of seeing and I was excited to have caught his bug. For a short while I saw the world through different eyes.

The initial enchantment with *Les Parapluies* quite quickly expanded into an obsession with anything by Renoir. I collected postcards of his paintings regardless of their painterly merit. At one stage I imagined having postcards of every painting he had done and I started making my own 'catalogue raisonné', sticking the postcards into a book of thick cream pages and laboriously typing little labels with the titles and the names of the lucky owners. I stoutly defended those nudes and still-lives of flowers, which my family considered sentimental and garish, and in defiance stuck Renoir reproductions all over my bedroom walls, although I could see that some paintings were much more successful than others.

I started painting in oils to try and emulate the brushwork and palette of the *Master* and I would ask for tubes of 'Renoir blue' paint. It was as if, for a short but intense period, the only way I wished to look at the world was through Renoir's eyes. He painted seductive women and was himself seductive in his brush strokes and with his pink and blue palette. It was maybe the fleshiness and the multi-coloured skin of some of his nudes that repulsed my parents and yet attracted me to the idea of a less puritanical world where it might be acceptable to be admired for my own pale pinkness and fleshiness, neither of which I was happy about.

Renoir has frequently been criticized for his love of looking at women both dressed and undressed and he never denied that the female form gave him intense pleasure. 'I am content with the first draggle-tail that comes along, provided she has good firm buttocks and breast' (Vollard, 1936: 266). He also frequently said, as reported by his son Jean, that he never experienced anything deeply unless he was able to touch it (Renoir, 1962). Painting was for him a way of touching. As anyone knows who has been to a life drawing class, the pressure and movement of the pencil or charcoal or paint on paper is as if one is touching the model, finding his or her form and shape through line and brush. Renoir's delight in what he painted or *touched* was apparent to me then, and it made me aware of how crucial it is for an artist to love the physical aspect of the work.

The size of *Les Parapluies* was one of the first things I was aware of. It is almost six feet high and it appeared enormous to me. This size of canvas had traditionally been reserved for use by portrait artists or for set scenes from history or mythology. If an artist had chosen a large canvas, then the Paris Salon expected a serious subject. Renoir was the first artist to use these large canvases for more mundane subjects that he took from everyday life. His choices of subject matter and the manner in which they were painted tested the liberalism of the members of the Salon and his paintings were often rejected as being too 'domestic' for such a large scale. It was this so-called 'domesticity' which was so appealing to me, and which I felt I could relate to, and was one of the reasons why the Impressionists were so easy to love.

The Impressionists rejected the conventional painting of the late 19th century where the palette was a restrained one of greys and browns and blacks, and where detail and the moulding of figures was paramount. Instead they attempted to capture passing moments of light and shade and the ever-changing nature of the natural world. Painting for them was about individual expression, rather than about painting to suit a market, although Courbet believed that if the painters painted what they saw around them these pictures would actually appeal more to buyers than the traditional pictures about historical or moral situations. How the painter saw the world was what mattered. Monet and Renoir who frequently painted together produced widely different paintings of the same scene. 'The very idea of "the finished work" was a misconception; "finish" and "style" were equally to be deplored ... "Two strokes might do the trick", as Renoir suggested: more precisely, two tones in juxtaposition, provided they were the right ones' (Danchev, 2012: 1338). The use of minimal strokes of paint was a very attractive idea. Maybe, I thought, if an effect could be conveyed so easily I would be able to emulate this myself. It seemed I didn't need to be able to draw if all it took was a couple of strokes of paint. I tried painting my own impressions of things, placing strokes of green paint against grey, or dabbing a point of red to signify a poppy, but at best these experiments looked like unappealing minestrone soup and conveyed nothing like the effects of light I was aiming for. How was it that a blob or line of intense blue next to a line of zinc white could so perfectly describe a bow on a dress, or a cloudy sky? It seemed extraordinary to me that so much could be expressed with so little. I could feel the painter's brush stroke and pressure and the emotions behind it as I made my own failed attempts to emulate his work. These body experiences were probably some of my first experiences of using myself as a sounding board for the other. In this case not a person but a work of art.

In the mid-19th century this impressionistic way of painting was viewed as naked exhibitionism by the art establishment and far too emotional and personal. The Salon regulars were used to having their artists' internal world of thoughts and feelings filtered through a conventional framework, where they were protected from having to think too much about the individuality of the artists. As a result the majority of Parisians found this new art both uncomfortable and unacceptable.

In this febrile climate Manet decided to risk even more and in 1863 he painted *Le Dejeuner sur l'herbe*, with a naked woman sitting in the countryside accompanied by two clothed men. It was considered outrageous that she was naked in an outdoor setting but, more importantly, it was the fact that she was neither embarrassed about her nakedness nor was she averting her gaze, but directing it instead out of the picture directly at the viewer. She was staring out of the painting and inviting an audience to stare back. This was far too provocative for the Paris of Napoleon III. Manet, though, was not put off and two years later he painted *Olympia*, his naked, prone prostitute with a tiny black bow round her neck and dangling her slipper off the couch. She is staring cynically out at us and daring us to stare back. In this new art the beholder was being acknowledged as a presence and being invited in.

I returned many times to the National Gallery with my parents and always ended up staring at *Les Parapluies*. Staring at people was considered rude and seemed to embarrass my parents if I indulged in it. But in the gallery I was delighted that I could stare without reproach, as it seemed that staring at paintings was to be welcomed. This was a heady idea; not only could I be part of this picture in my fantasies, but I was also being encouraged to look in this intense way. Although I was quite young and naïve at the age of ten, I don't think it is fanciful to think that staring at *Les Parapluies* and being stared at back, by the young woman and the girl in the picture, was my first benign experience of what being gazed at might entail; if I was fascinated by looking at others, they might also be fascinated by looking at me, and that might have a positive aspect. I had often become very uncomfortable when I was stared at in school, as I did not know what was being thought and I always feared criticism or rejection. Being stared at can be unnerving because we do not know what the other person is thinking. Yet staring is also an expression of a desire for more knowledge. It is a drive towards information about and connection with another. I wanted to know about and be known by another and it seemed that Renoir was encouraging me to do just that.

Renoir was often seen as a painter who reproduced the *male* gaze, but the critic Charles Harrison adds to this perception of the painter by including

> the beholder's share, our part in the interpretation and fashioning of the painting. … it also allows us to experience in imagination what it is like to both look and *be looked at* in this fashion. It is thus edifying for all of us, irrespective of the gender we think we start with.
> (Harrison, 2005: 35)

There is a lot of gazing going on in *Les Parapluies*. As well as the two figures looking out of the painting at me, the woman on the right, presumably the mother of the two girls, was looking down at her youngest daughter and the woman on the left was being gazed at by a man directly behind her. This young unaccompanied woman directed her gaze at me but she was also the object of an intense male gaze. Many of Renoir's paintings explore what it is like to look and be looked at in this way, whether we are male or female. The viewer inhabits a position from which they take part in the creative process of constructing the painting's meaning. We can be both the gazer and the gazed at.

The perfect place to indulge in the delights of this two-way process in the mid-19th century was at the theatre. The audience were not in darkness but lit up like the stage, so going to the theatre meant that you could stare at the audience and at the stage, using your opera glasses for both. I was delighted when I found a postcard of *La Loge* painted in 1874 (Figure 3.2).

The woman in the beautiful dress looked out from her box in the theatre directly at me and so I inevitably gazed back at her. The man behind her has his binoculars raised, so he is looking not at the stage but is gazing at

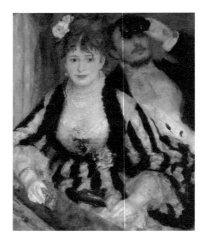

Figure 3.2 La Loge, Pierre-Auguste Renoir, oil on canvas, 1874.
© The Courtauld Gallery, London, UK/Bridgeman Images.

someone in the gallery. I felt his lack of attention allowed me to stare at his companion more myself. Renoir also painted *At the Theatre* in 1876 and *At the Concert* in 1880; two more paintings of women in boxes at the theatre, both of which found their way into my catalogue raisonne. Renoir was aware that this was not only a place where social status could be on display but also where relationships between men and women were highly visible. Here was a place where society could stare at itself. I was almost as enchanted with these three pictures as I was with *Les Parapluies*, because of the sense of drama and of being on show. Here was a life so unlike my own and which appeared to exude such confidence of status, many worlds away from the daily indignities that school presented me with and from which I longed to escape.

At the time, I was only aware of being encouraged to stare but now I can see that I was being encouraged to do more than that. I was staring at the female figures, measuring them, assessing them, and then it was as if I was metabolised in front of the canvas by those very figures who then seemed to be staring back at me. Because I'd identified with the figures it was easy to jump across the space and inhabit their positions, to become them and to stare back out of the canvas at my 20th-century self. I became the painting. At the age of ten I could slip seamlessly between the two positions, something that I found became more difficult as I got older.

Self-consciousness on the artist's behalf about the beholder has in the 21st century moved into another realm and become an integral part of our appreciation and understanding of art. As beholders of contemporary artistic works we know that we are necessary in bringing the work into being. Damien Hirst's pickled shark, *The Physical Impossibility of Death in the Mind of Someone Living*, requires *us* to make meaning and to put the title and the shark together to form an idea, to help the artist out. Without us the work is meaningless. Many contemporary artists presume that the audience is now a party to the self-consciousness of this exchange; it is what the art requires from us and that exchange has become essential to the act of looking. The relationship between the art and the beholder has in the 21st century moved into a different sphere.

As a ten-year-old I was not yet aware of the power I might hold as the gazer and how that role might develop and be more self-consciously constructed in the future by contemporary artists. The years when I was deeply in love with Renoir were years of transition for me. I was beginning to find a nascent sense of power and sense of self, both of which were helped by feeling that the artist needed me to gaze. This narcissistic fantasy that I was needed allowed me to engage with the process of how to really look at paintings and simultaneously encouraged me to think about how my own reactions were an essential part of that process. The idea that what I felt emotionally when looking at a painting might actually tell me more about the work was still in an embryonic stage – a process that was to be fully explored when I trained as a therapist. However it did seem to me at that time that art was about encountering other people's views and experiences of the world and thereby seeing the world and myself more clearly.

Chapter 4

Red paint

By the time I was in secondary school I had stopped seeing the world through a blue filter and was somewhat disdainful of Renoir prettiness. I was fifteen, permanently hungry and fractious at anything and everything. I was becoming cynical about my education, which still bored me. I looked for painterly interest outside of school. I needed to be introduced to an artist who might reflect something of my own teenage angst. The opportunity came on a family holiday in France.

This holiday, like many before it, entailed a great deal of camping. Camping had enabled our family to have a series of sometimes damp, sometimes exhausting holidays in Britain and on the Continent. This time at least we would have a permanent home for ten days in a converted sheep pen in the South of France. But we still had to get there. Our camper van was a precociously named VW Caravette. If I sat in the front on the bench seat I could watch the road and look down on the surrounding cars. But this was a much-desired place by all the family, and turns had to be taken. Sitting in the back was far less entertaining, as we'd be surrounded by cooking gear and bedding, which we'd have to brace ourselves against to try and get comfortable.

All this stuff was a constant reminder of all the apparently necessary but tedious processes of putting up tents, blowing up air beds, cooking sausages, washing up plastic plates and constantly repacking the VW. When it was my turn to be in the back I'd try and make some space to lie on one of the benches and watch the rows of poplars streaming past the windows. I was at any one time delighted and annoyed by everything and by myself.

La Bergerie, the sheep pen where we thankfully stayed after five days of driving, was close to the Provencal town of Vence. Here we had a murky weed-infested pool, a wonderful terrace overlooking a view down the valley, a kitchen of sorts and a working bathroom. I thought it luxurious. I spent one boiling afternoon on the terrace in a sunhat and shorts painting the view through the cypresses of the house next door, oblivious to everything except what I was looking at. I made a little green-grey oil painting, a Monet-Pissarro hybrid, or so I thought, which delighted and surprised me, as if it had come into being without any effort on my part.

On an oppressively hot and dusty day we visited the Chapel of the Rosary, which had been designed by Matisse for the Dominican sisters at Vence. Outside it was ninety degrees Fahrenheit, but inside the white chapel it was cool and quiet. We were the only visitors. We were allowed in by the nuns with strict instructions to be quiet and to cover up. Affronted at the gender-specific rules, I wrote in my holiday diary: 'They allow the public to see it on the certain condition that women were to be properly dressed. Of course men did not matter!' It was one of the simplest architectural spaces I had ever walked into. Blue and green light from the stained-glass windows flowed across the white tiles onto the floor and walls. The strange hieroglyphics of the Stations of the Cross, which were painted on the wall tiles in black paint, looked as if they had been sketched in a flurry of enthusiasm and terror, whilst the drawing of Mary with child was done with a few easy flowing lines. The chapel had the feel of an artist's studio and it was as if Matisse had just walked out.

All the annoyances about myself dissipated in this enclosed haven. For my young tumultuous and agnostic self, being in the chapel was a powerful spiritual experience, brought about by the shape, textures and cloistered air of the building. What looked from the outside like an empty white box was filled inside with the contents of the artist's imagination, both sublime and tortured. Matisse the atheist had created a space that reverberated with light, colour and silence. My body responded to this meditative building with a desire to lie down on the floor and relax, although the black and white tile drawings did seem edgy. In my diary I noted again: 'I thought Matisse could have put a little more thought into it' – a comment perhaps on the dissonance between the intense blue, green and yellow windows, and the sketchy black *Stations of the Cross* which I experienced as unformed. The building felt like a sanctuary for opposing feelings, both calming and discordant. I wondered whether the artist experienced the world as a mixture of these things. This was an appealing idea because it reflected my own confused state. The Chapel of the Rosary is one of the last works Matisse made and his only architectural project. He died three years after it was finished in 1954.

On our return from France I started to track down all I could about this newly discovered artist. Everything about Matisse excited me, from his drawings and his sculpture to his startling paintings. Quite early on in this quest I discovered *Woman Reading*, a small oil painting made when he was only twenty-five. The picture is of a dark interior with a woman sitting in a chair with her back to us.

We can just see a hint of the book that she is looking at. The painting made me think of those occasions in my own home when our sitting room became a warm enclosing place where I could lose myself in a book. I felt unkempt and fractious as a teenager and simultaneously longed for and fought against my need for containment. I didn't identify with the woman but I recognised the atmosphere Matisse had created, the warm brown and green space, lit by two lights, which gave off an aura of concentrated stillness. When I look at the painting now it evokes the 18th-century French painter Chardin or the Dutch Masters, but significantly for me then, it was the contained domestic interior which impressed me, and which, I was to discover, was what continued to absorb Matisse throughout his life.

The chapel at Vence, designed at the end of a long life, is a concrete example of what constructed spaces meant to Matisse. On that first visit I had picked up a certain tension and the feeling that, for Matisse, containment was not necessarily straightforward. The black and white painted tiles made me feel uncomfortable, but it was to be a long while before I had any idea of what that dissonance might be about and how it informed the artist's fascination with painting interiors.

Whilst still at school I came across a startling Matisse that cemented my connection to this artist and finally dissolved my ties to Renoir. It was *Red Studio*, or rather a good reproduction of it in a modern art magazine, and I cut it out and stuck it on my bedroom wall. I felt it was the most daringly different painting I had yet seen. It initially appeared to have little form, but it radiated colour. It reminded me of the red texture of a wool duffle coat my mother had made me when I was four. This coat had a hood with four toggles down the front and a cream brushed-cotton lining, which was printed all over with tiny red elephants. When given this coat I remember feeling completely understood. A few years later I was given a vibrant red paint box, which I treasured specifically because of its unique red colour. I didn't usually respond to or particularly like red, but it was this tomato soup redness with an undertone of yellow that seemed to have a physical effect on me. It was as if only this tone of red was right, as mostly reds were too infused with pink or orange to interest me. I had sometimes searched for this redness of the coat and paint box, hoping to find it replicated in another object, but I would very rarely find the exact tone which my body seemed to respond to, that is until I discovered *Red Studio* (Figure 4.1).

This re-igniting of my visual experiences from childhood was inseparable from the emotional responses generated at the time. The colour and the feeling were one and the same thing, and seeing the colour brought back the memories of those other objects and the delicious feelings associated with them. Colour and feelings are tightly bound together as the psychoanalyst Marion Milner discovered in her book of self-exploration, *On Not Being Able to Paint* (Milner, 1957: 157).

For me, this special red was an experience of longing, that had been met in the form of a little hooded coat and later by a tin paint box. Both had been objects that I had received at exactly the right time, perfect objects of desire. The reproduction of *Red Studio* re-awakened those feelings of intense childhood pleasure at the occasional but almost painful rightness of receiving a present that was previously not known about but is then

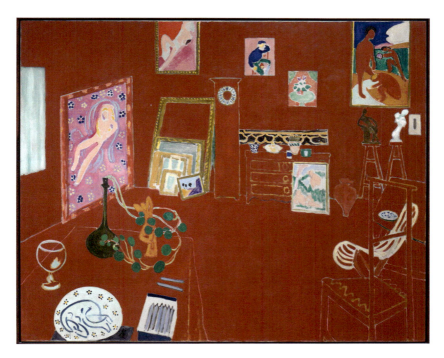

Figure 4.1 *The Red Studio*, Issy-les-Moulineaux. Henri Matisse, 1911. Mrs Simon Guggenheim Fund, The Museum of Modern Art, New York.
© photo SCALA, Florence.

immediately recognised as desired. So the first thing that the reproduction of *Red Studio* did was to envelop me in a sense of being seen and understood, and that was many years before I saw the actual canvas.

The redness of *Red Studio* is a thick flat Venetian red that seems to cover almost everything. There are no windows in the painting, although at first glance the pictures on the walls look like openings out of this claustrophobic space. The only perspective, apart from a thin yellow line around the edge of the room, is given by the objects themselves, which appear to float in thick tomato soup. The painting drew me into its space by making me look for signs of perspective. The yellow line might denote where wall becomes floor, or edge becomes table, but by the time I had noticed or questioned the lines I was there in the room and overwhelmed with red. Objects and paintings floated and yet they also appeared to be anchored, to know their place. At the centre of the picture there is a large void of redness, which drew my eye up and into this charged interior. The Danish painter Ernst Goldsmidt saw this painting on the wall in Matisse's studio and later recounted what Matisse had said: "'You're looking for the red wall", Matisse said to me … "That wall simply doesn't exist. Where I got that red from I simply couldn't say"' (D'Alessandro & Edenfield, 2010: 112).

Each object in the room seemed to me to carry an intense charge, as if they were not just treasured for their shape and colour but also for the importance to the painter himself. The crayons or pencils on the table were asking to be picked up and used. The empty wine glass has just been drained. The bamboo chair was expecting to be sat on by a model. The tendrils of a houseplant were lovingly draped over a small sculpture, as if they were both patiently expecting to appear on the next canvas. But the main objects in the studio were the paintings themselves, all ones, I discovered, that were painted by the artist. They were, from left to right along the back wall, *Large Nude* 1911, later destroyed, *Nude* 1909, *Corsican Landscape* 1898, *The Young Sailor II* 1906, *Purple Cyclamen* 1911, *Nymph and Faun* 1909, *Le Luxe II* 1907. The two sculptures on the right, the terracotta urn on the floor, and the chairs and table were all part of the environment of the studio during that period. I was thrilled by this privileged peek into Matisse's working space, and specifically by the autobiographical nature of the canvas. It showed me how important spaces and objects were to the painter, not just because of their visual delights, but also because of how they contained and held his world together. Later when I set up my own therapeutic consulting room, the positioning of the furniture and the objects I chose were crucial to my feeling of being held in the space and therefore being able to contain others.

For fifteen years I only saw *Red Studio* in reproduction and I always had the same intense reaction of love, brought about initially by my feeling response to *that red*, but also because of the sense that this was a painting about the painter himself. There was a *rightness* about the painting, as if it depicted sufficiency, although when I look at the painting now from a different perspective, *sufficiency* feels like entirely the wrong word for the jumble of pictures, furniture, sculptures and objects that hang in that redness.

When I finally saw the actual canvas of *Red Studio* in the 1980s, it had been brought over from The Museum of Modern Art in New York for a small exhibition at the National Gallery. The painting is large and of an unusual shape. It is almost 6ft high by just over 7ft wide, almost square in fact. There was nowhere to sit in front of the painting so I eventually sat on the floor unable to tear myself away. That special redness, which I had grown used to in my small reproduction, was both deeper and more lustrous than I could have imagined. It was still the red of my coat and paint box but more alive and intense. I got as close as I was able to the canvas. How had Matisse made this redness? It seemed unfathomable to me to have been able to make this depth of colour, which seemed to be beyond the normal capacity of red paint. It was as if it was operating outside my usual visual frame and beyond its own chemical properties.

The nature of the redness of *Red Studio* is exhilarating. The painting transmits this shade and tone of red with a confidence that makes it appear to be absolutely the right colour to describe this corner of the artist's studio. He may indeed not have known where that red came from, but I felt that Matisse had somehow painted his own emotional state. He was responding to his studio as if the painting was about both the confluence and the conflict between his inner and outer worlds, which he was struggling to bring together. 'What I am looking for is an interplay of colour that causes my emotion', he told Françoise Gilot, the artist, author and muse to Picasso (Gilot, 1990: 24).

The world of the studio is the well-known disorganised calm of Matisse's working space, and his internal emotional state is affected by the energized chaos of his unconscious life. *Red Studio* is an enormously energetic work about the act of painting and about the energy, love and struggle involved. The actual studio is a beloved place that houses the artist's work and reflects back to him how he sees the world. The metaphorical studio is also a creative container but an internal space where emotions jostle for recognition and release. Creativity is not a tidy activity for Matisse, but rather an erratic force with an energy all of its own which can spill out all over the place and *Red Studio* is certainly not a calm painting. The *rightness* is what I had experienced as a teenager, but I may have also unconsciously picked up on the ferment below the surface and simply dismissed it as my own.

When I look at *Red Studio* now I see a painting that has come out of a thunderstorm of feelings. It is as if the painting was made in such a state of emotional intensity that it can only just be contained by the edges of the canvas; as if the walls, paintings and objects might disengage from the canvas altogether. The artist and art therapist David Maclagan understands the unstable nature of this process: 'For the 'artist' on a high-wire in a circus, the greater the danger, analogous to involvement, the greater the need for control' (Maclagan, 2001: 139). My response to this instability is one of excitement touched with an edge of anxiety. How is it possible to contain the energy that the painted objects and art works generate in this red room? Each time I have managed to see the canvas I have been aware of a concern that this time the work might in some way have been interfered with or watered down, as if a work this intense might not be allowed to exist, that it would be 'too much' for some unidentified person. I suspect that this feeling may come partly from my own experiences growing up in a supportive but emotionally rather contained family; that the censorship that I feared would affect the painting was actually my own that I had absorbed from my early life.

Matisse struggled to contain and to paint his feelings, and then when he succeeded, he often found it hard to look at what he had made. 'There was a time when I never left my paintings hanging on the wall because they reminded me of moments of over-excitement and I did not like to see them when I had again become calm' (Matisse, 1908: 48). The painter as creator, just like the viewer, can be affected and then re-infected by his own work. If a painting works well it gains material qualities all of its own and can then turn its light back onto the artist where it has the ability to disturb with its own powerful energy. *Red Studio* is a painting of hyper-stimulation, which is then picked up by the beholder. The art historian James Elkins depicts this place of stimulation as an in-between territory and a place where boundaries dissolve. 'More than any other art, painting expresses the place between rule and ruthlessness in which we all find ourselves' (Elkins, 1999: 180). This is a disturbing place but also a highly creative one, and something that I would only begin to really understand when I became a psychotherapist (Miller, 2008: 13).

I found that when I gazed at *Red Studio* for long enough I began to feel as if my eyes and my brain were overloaded with redness and that this redness then had its own emotional affect. This use of colour to depict emotion is similar to the experience of synaesthesia, a neurological condition where feelings or words can be experienced as colours. The stimulation of one sensory pathway leads to an involuntary experience in a second sensory or cognitive pathway. It is as if pathways in the brain sometimes crossover and inadvertently stimulate each other. A singer I worked with later in life who had synaesthesia expressed her difficulty in managing the overstimulation she experienced when singing on stage. She was bombarded with visual as well as aural stimuli.

As far as I know no one has suggested that what Matisse experienced was synaesthesia, but his ability to convey his own emotional states through colour suggests that he could convert his feeling experiences into visual representations, something that the American painter Mark Rothko did with his enormous blocks of colour and the English painter Howard Hodgkin would also refine half a century later. Because of the non-representational nature of their paintings, both these modern artists require the beholder to spend time looking at and absorbing their work, until a feeling response is generated. This is also true of Matisse, yet his work is often viewed simply as one of decorative surfaces rather than of depth, so he may not always have elicited such intense looking.

Matisse painted the *Red Studio* when he was forty-two in 1911. At the beginning of that year he had spent a couple of months away from his family in Spain. He was hoping that the Spanish climate and the light would help him with his chronic insomnia and anxiety. He needed peace and intense light. He was becoming immersed in colour and experimenting with how blocks of colour can by themselves give depth and shape without a drawn perspective. He was abandoning obvious approaches to perspective and experimenting with representing his feelings in paint. He was no longer interested in an impression of what he saw (his view of the Impressionists was that they did not go far enough), but rather in an attempt to put on canvas what he felt about what he saw. 'An artist ... should not copy the walls, or the objects on a table, but he should, above all, express a vision of colour, the harmony of which corresponds to his feeling' (Flam, 1973: 51). It was as if paint could no longer convey how the painter's eyes saw the world but it also had to show how the internal could be pictured externally and integrated into what the eyes see. To try and bring these two together in paint required struggle and intense work.

During the time when I first became obsessed with Matisse he was seen mostly as a decorative painter of colour and light who was attracted to the surface of things. His paintings of odalisques surrounded by Algerian and Moroccan materials and highly decorated carpets persuaded much of the art world that this was a painter who was interested in depicting the beautiful and the exotic. His work was reproduced in posters and postcards and on carrier bags as a form of sophisticated graphics. As I became more engaged with the painter I found that my opinion – that there was more going on under the surface than this – was difficult to uphold. There seemed to be few art historians who understood Matisse as a painter of the emotional aesthetic or even those who seemed to feel deeply about his work. It wasn't until the writer Hilary Spurling published her two-part biography of Matisse that I felt that my responses to Matisse had been acknowledged (Spurling, 1998, 2005).

Spurling tackles the assumption that Matisse was simply a decorative artist and presents a compelling case of a man who felt haunted all his life by his decision to become a painter rather than the lawyer that his father had wished for. He walked a precarious line trying to keep a balance between his highly sensitized and sensitive psyche, which was easily overtaxed, and the anger and rage that would erupt when he was trying to work. He needed to harness this anger in order to be creative. Creativity was not a benign force for the artist but a battleground. A superficial viewing of his work might see it as charming or delightful but underneath this is a ferment of emotions, a thinly disguised struggle with the unconscious forces that he unleashes and then has to tame in his attempt to get his feelings about the visual world onto canvas.

The dramatic nature of his colours and the angularity of some of his portraits were viewed as strange in the early part of the 20th century. Between about 1904 and 1908 Matisse and the painter Derain represented the short-lived movement of *Les Fauves*, or *Wild Beasts*, so named to illustrate the violence of colour and brush strokes they used. Françoise Gilot, in her memoir about Matisse and Picasso, referred indirectly to Fauvism by naming these forces that Matisse struggled with.

> How difficult it must have been to face the wild beasts from within before unleashing their untamed energy onto the canvas, to uncover this savage self heretofore hidden under the veneer of reason and civilisation.
>
> (Gilot, 1990: 60)

I recognized this combination of sensitivity and rage in myself, characteristics which in my teenage years I had no idea how to harness or bring together. I wanted to be the brave young feminist who was not affected by her own feelings of shame and inadequacy, or by the criticisms of others. Instead I struggled to find a place where I could fit in and conform, whilst my fury about feeling that I had to do this bubbled up underneath, and then expressed itself as boredom and rage. When I finally came across 'the wild beasts' I could see why Matisse's expressive aesthetic had so appealed to me and that *Red Studio* was a synthesis of those intense feelings. The painting managed to create a place where desire and execution came together and as a result expressed the prize of the creative struggle.

I have relished *Red Studio* ever since I first put that reproduction on my wall and I return to it often when I feel lacking in creative energy. My appreciation of the painting has also grown with me, from that early thrill of recognizing the colour as a part of my own history, to my present admiration of the painter who struggled with internal daemons in a bid to get his emotional life onto the canvas, and in so doing conveyed the extreme tensions involved in creativity. Matisse introduced me to the realization that making art was a wrestling match between the desire to convey colour and form, and the unconscious emotions that might be stirred up by this process. He showed me that painting communicated on both conscious and unconscious levels, and that the subterranean world stirred up by the making of and then the looking at art was where the excitement was – an insight that informed my work later when in the consulting room.

Chapter 5

Stillness

The *wild beasts* of my teenage years became more quiescent as I prepared to go to university. Life seemed to be opening up and I was less fractious with my lot. I had chosen one of the new universities, which were starting up in the 1960s, in a deliberate attempt to break away from my rigid and unimaginative girls school. The University of Kent wanted five hundred students who had enough energy and enthusiasm to get a campus going. The tutors were less interested, at that point, in our academic potential, and I was delighted to be joining an experiment, the intention of which was to bring about a metamorphosis on a muddy patch of land above Canterbury. In the spring I was interviewed in an old farm building in the middle of a field and told that by October there would be a finished college building where we could live and be taught. I felt that I was wanted and might even have something to offer. Although excited by this prospect and by the idea of leaving school, I was also fearful and I needed a holiday from which calm plateau I could contemplate this brave new world.

During that summer my brother and I joined up with ten friends and rented a villa in Tuscany. It was a large square slightly dilapidated building in the formal garden of an imposing house. We had lots of bedrooms, an enormous kitchen and a glorious shady terrace. From here we could look down on an ancient landscape of small rounded hills and groves of ash-grey olive trees, interrupted by sentinel-like cypresses and the occasional crumbling stone hut. I felt that I had been transported back into the 15th century. It was a very hot August and the scent of thyme pervaded the terrace. Here we talked, read and fell in and out of love with each other. In the evenings we retreated from the mosquitoes into the kitchen and ate pasta and peaches. I spent my time taking photos of our friends who were already at university, and who through my eighteen-year-old eyes appeared astoundingly intelligent and fascinating. After a while they got used to me pointing the camera at them whilst they ate, talked, read and drew each other. Using my camera as a protection from these beautiful creatures, I inhabited the position of the one who could gaze.

One of my brother's intentions on this holiday was to see as many of the Piero della Francesca paintings he had on his bedroom walls as he could.

Looking out from our terrace it was as if I was in my brother's bedroom at home; these hills and cypresses and delicate dark green trees seemed exactly as the artist had painted them, the pale hot light casting shadows on the terraces. Our villa was close to the area of Sansepolcro, where the painter had lived and worked for a lot of his life and where many of his frescoes were still in their original buildings. Now many of these beautiful works have been moved to museums where air conditioning and artificial lights have protected them but destroyed the spirit of place. When we were there however the art had not yet been wrenched out of its context.

Our terrace view reminded me of della Francesca's paintings in the National Gallery when, on family visits to see the Impressionists, we had sometimes veered off into the rooms of the early Italians and looked at the three magnificent canvases of the Renaissance artist that the gallery owned. The painting of *St Michael The Archangel* didn't particularly interest me; I found his combination of wings and armour a bit confusing, although I did like his little red boots. However *The Baptism of Christ*, with the dove, wings outstretched, hovering above Christ's head and the three angels standing barefoot on the grass watching John pouring the water, delighted me with its symmetry. The glimpses of the Italian landscape with its soft muted colours felt exotic to my English eyes. I imagined that the angels were whispering to each other about their own affairs, their attention only half taken up by the baptism happening in front of them. They had such ordinary round human faces, with no trace of ethereal spirituality and I loved their earthiness. They looked like three curly-haired young women who had just happened upon this scene by a river in the Tuscan landscape. I was unaware that they were probably men, but despite my own lack of a religious upbringing the painting felt accessible to me in ways in which many overtly religious paintings did not. This painting was about ordinary people.

It was the painting of *The Nativity* (Figure 5.1) in the National Gallery that I knew best however, as it had been co-opted into our family in a rather odd way. My mother had decided one Christmas, completely against our normal secular holiday routine, to make a three-dimensional replica of della Francesca's painting out of clay.

She did not manage to recreate the entire painting; there was no tree-studded Italian landscape in the background, but the sloping roof and precarious wall of the manger were, I think, made out of cardboard. The main figures were all made in clay and then painted. The angels were modelled in one piece with a mass of conjoined hair, flowing gowns and lutes, and the pale slightly washed-out tones of della Francesca's palette were carefully copied and painted on in watercolours. Mary's blue cloak flowed around her knees and a pale cream clay baby lay on top of it. The two shepherds had rather unformed faces, as the details in the painting were no longer there to be copied; either the artist had not finished them, or the

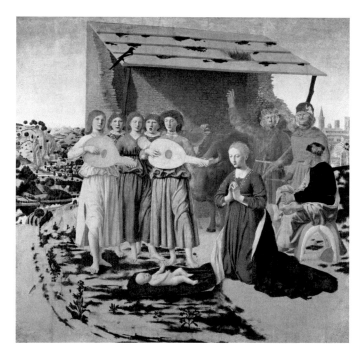

Figure 5.1 Nativity, Piero della Francesca, tempera on panel, 1470–1475.
© National Gallery London, UK/Bridgeman Images.

paint had been removed when it was cleaned. But the two faceless men stood in the background regardless and it seemed not to matter. Joseph sat sideways on his stool in detached contemplation. There was no sign of the donkey or the ox, which are rather thin and flat in the painting and would, I imagine, have been more difficult to model. My mother was far more interested in the formal composition of the figures, how they held together in groups, and in the delicious understated colours. The simplicity and the painting's relative lack of Christian iconography also probably appealed to her. The whole conceit of the clay model seemed to work as long as you didn't look at it sideways or from behind, in which case the artifice crumbled at the sight of unpainted grey lumps. 'The crib', as it was called, was brought out for a few years at Christmas time – more in honour of the artist than of Jesus – until its dusty, flaky appearance was too much for all the family and it subsequently disappeared permanently into a cupboard.

This strange three-dimensional exercise showed me how della Francesca used perspective and depth and how all his figures interconnected with each other. I was told that, just prior to the period when the artist was working, the scientific applications of perspective had been discovered and that this aspect of drawing was seen as an interplay between art and science; a coming together of the two disciplines. *On Perspective in Painting* was the artist's major written work, in which he explored the new ideas around perspective (Della Francesca, 1474–1482). By sculpting the painting my mother had laid open its simple but effective structure, a careful balance of forms against background. I was also touched by the way she had tried to emulate the delicacy of the painting of the faces by using a tiny brush to highlight the eyebrows and eyes of the figures. For anyone who knew the work it was obvious what these painted lumps of clay referenced. For those who didn't, it worked, just about, as a rather strange model of a Christmas crib.

With these images of the painter in mind, and away from the intensity of the burgeoning relationships taking place on the Italian terrace, some of us made trips into the surrounding towns to search out buildings and paintings. On one of these trips my brother and I went off on a Piero hunt to look for the chapel that housed the *Madonna del Parto* in the small town of Monterchi (see Figure 5.2). We eventually found the tiny chapel in the middle of a field. It was lunchtime, there was no one about and the door was padlocked. It seemed an unlikely place for the fresco but a guidebook assured us we were in the right place. Eventually a local farmer saw us sitting on a wall, opened up the chapel for us and left us to it.

It was as if the Madonna had been waiting for us to arrive. Two angels were in the process of drawing back the curtains of the tent she was standing under, showing her off to her small audience. She stood resplendently with her right hand resting on her rounded belly. Her blue dress was unbuttoned where her pregnancy was at its fullest. Maybe she was about to open her dress to show us her belly. Her gesture seemed both enticing and intimate and I imagined she would have no shame if we were to see her naked. Her hair was plaited and tied with ribbons and her halo rested on her head like a fashionable flat hat. She looked out at us from a calm white face full of composure. It was a sister face to Mary's in *The Nativity* in London, although this Madonna's hooded eyes had the inward-looking expression of a woman at full term. The pale blues, greens and pink paint were a more washed-out version of the ones I knew from the National Gallery paintings, but here, instead of hanging framed in gold leaf, the colours blended into the stone walls of the chapel. The angels were painted as smaller reduced figures, and by standing there in their stockinged feet they emphasized the Madonna's stature, which appeared almost gargantuan, as if to underline her importance. Despite this sense of performance it felt like a simple domestic scene, as if we were being shown Mary in a relaxed moment at home. The atmosphere of intimacy was enhanced for me by my brother and I being the only two people in the chapel, and by the fact that

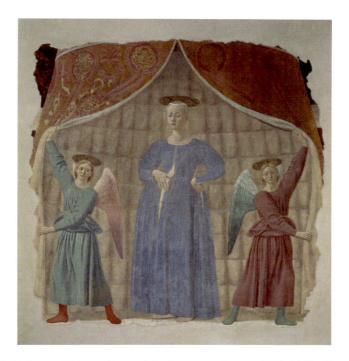

Figure 5.2 Madonna del Parto, Piero della Francesca, fresco, 1450–1470. Chapel of the Cemetery, Monterchi.
© Italy Bridgeman Images.

it had been specially opened up for us, as if we had indeed come to visit the Madonna herself.

In the 1990s the fresco was rehoused in a special museum in town and I wonder whether in its new abode it now evokes this same intimate atmosphere. I have no desire to visit it again, wrenched as it has been from its womb-like home. Art historians think that the original chapel was used by pregnant women who brought thanks to the shrine for their conceptions, and also by women who longed to be pregnant in the hope that the Madonna would help them. The *Madonna del Parto* certainly looked as if she was party to a powerful female mystery. If I had known then that I would some years later have had my own difficulties with conceiving, I might well have offered her some flowers.

This time alone with the Madonna impressed on me the humanity and the importance of the stillness of the moment in della Francesca's work. Despite her stature and imposing presence this Mary was an ordinary woman who had been drawn into an extraordinary story. There was no fancy artifice here. Even the angels looked like indeterminate male/female peasants in their rough wool clothes and knitted socks. It was as if the artist was saying: *this is how things are, and if you look long enough you can become part of this too; miracles can happen to you*, or even, with a further stretch of the imagination, he might be suggesting that *being alive and human is already a miracle*. The painting induced a meditative state in my brother and me. We sat on a rough bench for a long while staring at the fresco and loving how unlike it was to most of the Renaissance Madonnas we knew. There were no fanfares, no heavenly spirits, just a serene pregnant woman in a tiny chapel in the middle of the Tuscan countryside. Outside olive trees grew in profusion in the hot baked earth. I felt warmed into life by the fresco and excited about the new possibilities waiting for me in the autumn.

The town of Arezzo was the main port of call on our Piero tour. A group of us went one day to visit *The Legend of the True Cross* in the Basilica of San Francesco. Here in the middle of a small town and surrounded by other visitors the experience was far less intimate than it had been at Monterchi. In the central chapel there were three layers of frescos up the walls and covering the ceiling. The effect was overwhelming as there were so many paintings to look at and each one told a different part of the story. I leant my head against the wall as I tried to follow the images of how wood from the Garden of Eden had been made into the cross of Christ's crucifixion. It seemed a long and complicated story and I gave up as the cumulative effect of the frescos took over.

Each level of fresco was busy with people, animals and action. The battle scene was an intense density of men and horses. Each sword, each raised arm, each helmet conveyed violence and brutality, the standards swayed across a pale blue sky. Sweaty hair stuck to faces, horses reared and gasped. The overall effect was powerful but it was the details that absorbed me. The individual faces of the warriors were painted with extreme delicacy. They showed fear, concentration and horror but each expression was unique. The horses too were painted as individuals. Their foaming gaping mouths and startled eyes conveyed a deep sensitivity to their individuality. Men and animals were all trying to free themselves from this dense mess of embattled bodies.

It was some of the smaller fresco panels and elements of the larger ones that delighted me the most. At the end of a long fresco named *The Reception of the Queen of Sheba by King Solomon* (Figure 5.3) I was very taken with the hindquarters of a horse. Two men were standing talking and one of them had his hand across the back of his white horse. The horse's head was hidden by the owner's hat but the horse's behind conveyed the character of the beast. It was a solid reliable animal, standing patiently by its owner and waiting. Beyond the white horse was the head of a black horse, neighing and showing its enormous white teeth. This horse was more aware than the two men were of the important scene unfolding beside them all, as a group of devout women bent their heads in prayer.

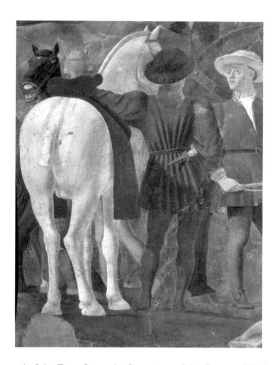

Figure 5.3 The Legend of the True Cross, the Reception of the Queen of Sheba by King Solomon, detail of two horsemen, Piero della Francesca, fresco, completed 1464, Arezzo, Italy.
Photo © Raffaello Bencini/Bridgeman Images.

The men, absorbed in their conversation, were taking little notice of anything else. Beyond them I could glimpse a hilly landscape, very like the one we could see from our terrace. There was a remarkable stillness in this fresco as if the air was without movement and, even though the men and the neighing horse might be making sounds, the painter seemed to have silenced them in their tracks. This was how the world was in this moment of time for these people and these animals, absorbed in their daily thoughts. The painter had again juxtaposed the ordinary next to the miraculous; his horsemen were not cyphers for the religious story but two individuals who just happened to be there whilst the religious mystery unfolded around them. For these two men, whatever was happening around them, there was time for contemplation.

I could now see more of what had appealed to my mother in her modelling of *The Nativity*. I felt that she had recognized something universal in the structure of the figures and the way they connected to the landscape.

This universality had its roots in images that were around way before Christianity, and came from a deep humanity and love of people and animals. The artist's work went far beyond religious iconography to depict the state of being human in the 15th century. It was probably the first time I understood something about how art can be informed by the landscape and culture in which the artist lives, as if these things are in the artist's bones, without him necessarily realizing it. The paintings still convey to me a deep sense of belonging and since that trip I have continued to equate della Francesca with the countryside of Italy as if there could never be any separation between the two.

When the holiday was over and I got back to London, I blacked out the tiny bathroom window, put a board over the bath, set up my enlarger and printed up my black and white photos. There were one or two prints of buildings but the majority were of the friends, sitting, standing and talking to each other with the view of hills and olives behind them. They seemed at ease with their bodies and unaware of my presence. There was a quality of warmth about these photos, as if the Italian landscape had embraced us in its liquid light, lowered our blood pressure and shown us how to be still. Back in the colder autumn light of London, the photos reminded me of the painter's frescos, silent contemplative people absorbed in the moment and unaware of anything that might be happening outside the frame, however monumental.

Since that hot initiatory and love-filled summer in Tuscany, no Renaissance painter has come close for me to Piero della Francesca's warmth, or that ability to paint all his figures, regardless of religious or work status, as straightforward human beings. That period of immersion in his work encouraged me to feel that my need for quiet and stillness had in some way been acknowledged. The painter had accentuated my own emerging need for introversion and contemplation, something that I was only just beginning to notice and understand. I had to accept that I responded to his work from a different part of me than that part excited by *Red Studio*. I began to think more about who I was or could be, and whether these different parts might be able to come together.

Much later when I had a therapy practice of my own, I would be reminded of Piero della Francesca's paintings when sitting with patients who were struggling with concern at their own introverted needs. They saw their exhaustion and need for quiet as a problem that didn't fit with an extraverted society. Some felt that they were failing to be like other people whom they said were constantly involved in energetic events and were 'at the centre of things where life happened'. Whilst suggesting that they might be mistaken, I would then find I had conjured up the *Madonna del Parto* quietly contemplating her own miracle, or the three angels chatting amongst themselves as Christ is baptized. The paintings helped me to hold the space for my patients, enabling them to stay with their stillness and provide the context for their own small miracles to happen.

Chapter 6
Touch

After university I perversely persuaded myself that I should forego a career in the visual arts and become a teacher instead. That idea soon crumbled beneath me and I thankfully gave up my teaching course and managed to get accepted by the BBC onto one of their training courses to become an assistant film editor. The film cutting rooms introduced me to a new partner and through him to a new circle of friends. One of the friends was a postgraduate student at Cambridge who invited us to stay with him in the city as long as we didn't mind sleeping on the sofa. But this was no ordinary sofa and no ordinary house. Our friend Alan was looking after Kettle's Yard for the art enthusiast Jim Ede. In the summer months Ede would leave his house in the charge of favoured students so that he could have a break from being constantly on call whenever someone rang the bell and wanted to see his collection. Before the house became famous and was opened as a museum, Ede believed in the principle of an open-door policy to anyone who was interested.

With Jim Ede safely away on holiday we were able to explore the house and the art collection and for two days harbour a belief that it was all ours. More important than the idea of possession, though, was the freedom to visit, revisit, sit in front of, draw and take photographs of the pictures and objects that engaged us. Occasionally visitors would knock on the door and interrupt our domain, but most of the time it felt as if we were in a hallowed place, where the noise of the world was shut out and we could tune in to the voices around us. Here I was surrounded by art and had the stillness I now craved.

Late on the first evening my partner and I became the sole occupants of the main gallery. We settled down on a low cream sofa, long enough to accommodate us both toe to toe. The idea of sharing the sofa surrounded by art was intoxicating. Alan had retreated to another part of the house having locked us in with dire warnings not to set off the burglar alarm. Any need for glasses of water or open windows had to be suppressed until he came to let us out in the morning. Late evening light filtered into the room from a high window, just enough for us to make out the shapes of bleached country wooden furniture and small sculptures on tables and ledges. I was delighted to be falling asleep in this room full of early 20th-century art.

During the night I woke up and wandered around in my bare feet, feeling my way on the wooden boards and hoping not to set off the burglar sensors. I had looked at the sculpture *Bird Swallowing a Fish* by Gaudier-Brzeska during the day and had been entranced by the violence and beauty of the work (see Figure 6.1). The thought that I could experience it entirely by myself was what had now woken me up. I remembered that it was on a piece of roughly sawn elm, and in the dark I could just make out the large open V of the outline of the sculpture. There was nothing to keep me away from the work, no frame or rope or obvious boundary, so I padded towards it and put my hands on it. I could feel the fatness of the overstuffed bird and the angularity of the rocket-like fish forcing open the bird's mouth. I didn't need to see it; touch was sufficient. My hands found both extremities of the piece at once. The tails of the combatants were raised up at either end and kept the sculpture beautifully balanced in the

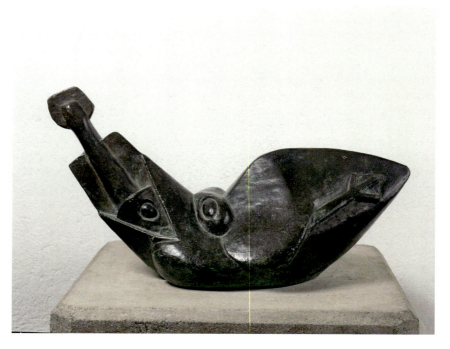

Figure 6.1 *Bird Swallowing a Fish*, Henri Gaudier-Brzeska, bronze, c.1960. Kettle's Yard, University of Cambridge.
© UK/Bridgeman Images.

middle at the base of the bird's neck as it craned its beak upwards. The tension between the two animals was what was keeping them rigid in this moment of contact. The fight that the fish and bird were engaged in was surely eventually going to be terminal for one of them, but it was not obvious who would survive. The bird's legs were stretched back along its body, its feet splayed out against its wings. I could feel the three toes pushing against its chest, trying to tense against the overlarge prey, which seemed to be boring into the bird's gullet. I put my finger on the fish and could feel the arrow-shaped form driving itself like a rocket into the bird's throat. The eyes of the fish and the eyes of the bird bulged under my fingers, popping out of their sockets in horror at their mutual dilemma. Both animals appeared to be victims and agents in this act of destructive piercing and swallowing. The work was at the same time both sharp and smooth; the phallic power and sexuality of the piece was conveyed through its mechanistic and aggressive angular edges and its rounded, fleshy fullness. The head of the fish was a triangle drilling into the bird's sharp-beaked open mouth and yet the body of the bird was plump and smooth. Under my fingers the surfaces of the sculpture felt very simple, as if this act of mutual destruction was straightforward and normal. I couldn't decide who was the assailant, was it the bird or the fish? They seemed equally matched and caught up in some ancient ritual of engorgement.

The sculpture was depicting what seemed like a violent act, but I could also sense the tenderness of the artist's touch, his intuitive understanding of his subject, and the expression of his own psychic engagement with the two animals. Although reduced to their essential elements each animal retained its intrinsic characteristics. This was not sloppy sentimentalism or an anthropomorphic re-invention; it was as if the artist had spent years watching birds over the sea and had synthesized the moment of attack into a few smooth bronze surfaces.

This bird and fish were related to birds and fishes of the past and represented all their ancestors. I felt that I was touching a sculpture that was made with an understanding about the atavistic nature of a relationship that goes back for millennia and that transcended time itself. I kept rolling my fingers over the surfaces as if, in the dark, I had come across an ancient artefact and was feeling my way into its shapes and meaning. I thought of the cave paintings of bison I had seen in France, which equally conveyed the symbiotic and long-standing relationship between animal and man, regardless of the passing centuries.

As I touched *Bird Swallowing a Fish* I could think of no better way of engaging with art. I was in the dark, it was warm in the gallery and completely quiet and I had the sculpture entirely to myself. It was an intensely private experience and mildly erotic, as if I was touching the body of the artist. This is the best that any encounter with art can be – a solitary experience far away from the usual people-filled gallery, allowing a focussing of senses deep into the intentions and meaning of a work. I wanted to continue feeling my way around the form for as long as my fingers spoke to me of what was under my hands.

What my hands felt was that Gaudier-Brzeska intuitively knew things about the innate and complex nature of animals, and the ways in which those complex natures are also true of humans; that we are bodies that bond and merge and copulate but that we are also capable of tearing each other apart. Sometimes it is difficult for us to separate the creativity from the destruction, the one from the other, just as I could not decide who was feeding or dismembering who, in the sculpture beneath my hands. I could feel the violence and tension from the sculpture transmitted through my body. Relying on my touch rather than on my eyesight seemed to have helped me to respond in this way. The three-dimensionality of the piece had required a haptic response. Maybe all three-dimensional work is best understood this way, through the fingers rather than the eyes.

I don't remember feeling guilty about touching the sculpture. In the 1970s touching sculpture was not considered to be so destructive to the materials as it is now, and the necessity of using my hands in the darkness seemed the best way then of connecting with the work. I always have a desire to touch sculpture, to help me to understand how the work was made, and with what kind of attention and what kind of marks. I feel I lose a lot by having to resist this in modern art galleries. What I had discovered by my touch in the dark was that not only did the sculpture speak to me, but also that I could respond and speak to the sculpture. I could feel and re-feel certain surfaces, almost as if I was learning them and memorizing them in my body. I could follow the cuts that the sculptor had made and in that way I could enter into this piece of bronze just as the work could enter into me. By getting used to the physical object it began to become part of me and to be incorporated into my sense of self. Much the same way as a musician might feel about their musical instrument, or a lover about a partner, it soon became difficult to tell where my body ended and the object began. This sense of fusing with a work of art allowed me to be open to new questions about the artist's intentions and the intense emotions that generated the shapes and marks he made.

This place where bodies communicate with bodies is the place where empathy begins. The sculptor Barbara Hepworth expressed this place as the source of her work: 'I rarely draw what I see. I draw what I feel in my body' (Hepworth, 1966: 11). We can know something in our bodies that we may not intellectually understand. My sense of Gaudier-Brzeska's intuition about the nature of the contact between the bird and the fish was enabled by his own empathy with his subjects, which was conveyed through his touch and then into his work. I was affected by this at the time on a visceral level but wasn't consciously aware of how it had happened. It intrigued me to think that it is not only the mind that can know but that the body can know too, in a different way. It began in me a questioning of the common, but actually rather strange, experience that we live with most of the time, that there is a rigid idea of a brain/body separation.

I became more immersed in this later in life when discovering how to intuit my patients better. When I became a therapist I became aware of how bodies can communicate feelings across space and of how to trust the reactions my body had to the movements in my patient's psyches. Sometimes I would feel a pain in my body before a patient was able to acknowledge it as theirs. Or my body would react violently to an unexpressed emotion in the room. Once my foot shot out as if to kick my patient who was struggling with her repressed anger. The anger was then available to be talked about. The body knows and understands in a different way than the mind does (Sidoli, 2000).

Eventually I began to get cold and crept across the gallery and negotiated my place back on the narrow couch, my feet finding two other feet to lodge against. I was acutely aware of my physicality as I lay in the dark, feeling again the planes, angles and curves that had captivated me with their tenderness and violence. I was still young and impressionable and felt that this artist had entered my psyche forcefully and unbidden. I identified with his youth and immense creativity. I found out many years later that after Gaudier-Brzeska had made this sculpture in 1914 he had then cast it, not in bronze but in gunmetal. This prescient casting was made a year before he was killed in action in France by a single bullet at the age of twenty-three; the same age that I was then.

Gaudier-Brzeska's brief but intense life was originally brought to public attention by Jim Ede's book *Savage Messiah*, which he published thirty years after the artist's death (Ede, 1971). The book is based mainly on the correspondence between Henri Gaudier and his companion, the Polish woman Sophie Brzeska, who was eighteen years older than him. Gaudier adopted her name to help ease the difficulty of sharing lodgings – they explained their relationship as that of brother and sister. The letters between them are full of intense desires to be creative, as well as expressions of narcissism and of mutual specialness. Much that has been written about the artist since then has carried forward the idea, originated in these letters, of a messianic genius who had an unconsummated love affair and then tragically lost his life in the First World War. The reputation of any artist of quality who dies prematurely young will suffer under the weight of unfulfilled expectations, and it is impossible to judge how Gaudier-Brzeska would have developed as a sculptor, but his legacy has been frozen into a story of a tragic genius. What Jim Ede's promotion of Gaudier-Brzeska did though was to bring his small body of work to international attention, and he is now recognized as one of the most important members of the European avant-garde who lost their lives to the First World War.

Upstairs in Kettle's Yard we discovered a small room full of drawings. They were of animals – cats, monkeys, cocks, stags, foxes and horses, drawings of nudes and wrestlers and portraits of his friends and acquaintances made in the few brief years of his artistic practice in London. Many were made with the thin tip of a stylus pen, the line flowing without interruption or hesitation, enveloping a form and turning it by some miracle of expectant vision into an apparently three-dimensional object.

About ten years after this initial introduction to the artist I visited a small London gallery to see an exhibition of his drawings. There was one of a horse and rider for sale, for the enormous amount of a thousand pounds. That was all the money I had in the world at the time and I talked myself out of buying it. I have regretted having that exciting and fluid drawing on my walls ever since.

Gaudier-Brzeska had no formal training. He was entirely self-taught and seemed to relish the challenges that his lack of classical technique presented him with. He had used sketchbooks since he was a child in France, although he destroyed many of these as he saw no purpose in them once he had mastered what he wished to master. When he arrived in England he made odd bits of money working in offices and then for a graphic designer, but soon gave up all paid work to concentrate on sculpture. He set himself tasks so that he could learn about working in three dimensions, beginning by working with clay and then moving on from modelling to cutting from stone. He began direct cutting into stone after visiting Jacob Epstein in his studio and being impressed and encouraged by him. Epstein had challenged the young man on that first meeting by asking whether he cut directly into stone. Gaudier-Brzeska had capitulated and then immediately went back to his studio and carved his first piece, believing that to be a real sculptor this is what he had to do.

He couldn't afford the stone or marble he needed and so begged and borrowed offcuts. He was hungry, angry, unkempt, smelly and immensely proud. He sometimes refused money for his work because he didn't want to be seen to be needy. His pride and arrogance meant that he was frequently half starved, but his fierce independence made him uninhibited and hence allowed him freedom to experiment with many techniques. As a result he produced innovative work whether it was modelled in clay, chiselled from stone or carved from a small bone toothbrush. Enid Bagnold, the novelist, said of the artist: 'Gaudier was like a dagger in the midst of us. He had a hungry face (we did not know how hungry) and a mind made of metal. He talked like a chisel and argued like a hammer' (Silber, 1996: 58).

Gaudier-Brzeska was an outsider and he used this position very self-consciously as a way of developing something that the British art establishment might have shied away from and been shocked by. His lack of concern about what others might think excited me, and his contradictory qualities of aggression and gentleness, of intense feeling and ribald humour, made me feel more comfortable with my own opposing desires for both excitement and quiet reflection. This ability to see the dark and the light at the same time, and to embrace both, seemed to be a more conscious and extravert expression of the struggle that Matisse had experienced.

Gaudier-Brzeska accepted the more aggressive part of his nature and used the energy of this to drive his work onwards. During the time of that visit to Kettle's Yard I was struggling with my first real job and trying to understand my place in the world as a woman. I frequently felt angry and frustrated by what I was experiencing as the misogyny and aggression shown towards women who refused to play their expected roles, yet I remained shy and frequently avoided confrontation. Working as an assistant film editor in the BBC was an unusual role for a woman at that time and a small group of us were subjected to sexism and subliminal attacks on our competence. I kept any ambition I had secret, but this made me feel stifled and unable to grow. It was obvious to me that men had a much easier time of it in the working world.

Gaudier-Brzeska appealed to my desire to lead a less inhibited life. He seemed able to express, without concern as to how he might be seen, both the violence and empathy that he recognized in himself and others. On the brink of the First World War he was beginning to explore the idea that one emotion cannot exist without the other, that they are both an essential part of being alive and that the dark and the light are two sides of a whole. Three years after the war ended, Jung published *Psychological Types* in which he introduced his ideas about this duality called enantiodromia, 'Construction and destruction, destruction and construction – this is the principle which governs all the cycles of natural life, from the smallest to the greatest' (Jung, 1971: para 708).

The drawings and sculptures that resulted from the artist's visits to wrestling bouts reflect this duality of feelings. They explore the powerful musculature of the wrestlers, the interlocking of two bodies and the tension between two foes waiting to physically engage; although the white bas-relief of *The Wrestlers* (Figure 6.2) that he carved in plaster seems more about a ritualistic and tender meeting between bodies and about a sensitivity of skin against skin. The relief suggests playfulness rather than aggression and the delights of touching and embracing another body. The men are naked and locked into a complicated and un-muscular hug.

The artist loved the physicality of moulding clay and chipping away at stone and the three-dimensionality of the work; a world of planes and forms was the world that he could experience through his hands. It was also in the creating of form that the sculptor explored his feelings about the world: 'I shall present my emotions by the arrangement of my surfaces; the planes and lines by which they are defined' (O'Keeffe, 2004: 293). This ability to express his emotions and his intense aesthetic experiences through

46 Touch

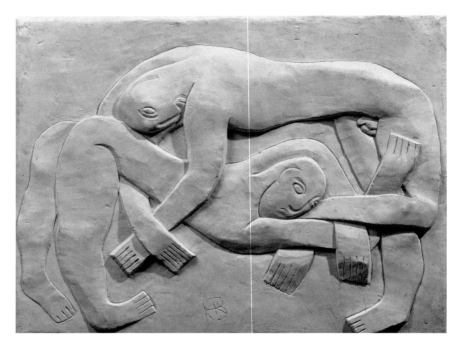

Figure 6.2 The Wrestlers, Henri Gaudier-Brzeska, herculite relief, 1965. Private Collection. © Christie's Images/Bridgeman Images.

form was picked up and experienced by me through my body and through touching, looking at and exploring shapes that had been made and directed by the artist's torrent of feelings.

With *Bird Swallowing a Fish* Gaudier-Brzeska introduced me to the idea that an art work can be the object through which two people can meet and experience each other. It can be a sensual and erotic experience or one that stirs up feelings of violence and destruction. The fascination that was kindled in me by that first visit to Kettle's Yard and being able to touch *Bird Swallowing a Fish* began an internal discussion in me about my own creative and destructive powers. Could there be a link between the two? It would be a while before I could look at this idea directly.

Chapter 7

Beads and threads

Whilst I was working in television my chances to look at any art slowly diminished. I had little spare time to spend away from the engaging process of learning about the visual language of moving images. I managed to work my way up from the cutting rooms and became a director of schools and children's programmes, and then eventually a freelance producer, directing documentaries for the newly formed Channel Four. Finally I was making films about issues that I cared about. It was hard work. I travelled abroad a lot and was under constant pressure from deadlines.

Early on in my television career I had been given an old Maasai necklace by a friend who had been in Tanzania for two years (Figure 7.1). This was a heavy circular object of predominately oval red beads with a few yellow, green and blue ones all threaded onto thick metal wires. Some of the rows were made from pieces of older necklaces, themselves made up of tiny beads and integrated into the whole. The wire used was rough hard wire, rusting in places. The necklace would have been one of many worn by a Maasai woman. She would have pulled it over her head where it would have rested on her shoulder blades and stuck out above her breasts.

The centre was too small for me to get it over my head and so I imagined that the woman would actually have been a girl, although when I later filmed the Maasai myself, I realized that all the women were smaller and slighter than me. I was delighted with this present, which when hung on the wall of my first house brought an exotic glamour to the sitting room.

The longer I lived with the necklace the more I felt that it wasn't just a piece of beaded craft-work but an art work in its own right. It affected me every time I caught sight of it and it always made me feel joyful. It seemed to transmit a powerful energy through its vibrant primary colours, its weighty presence (it needed a strong hook to hold it on the wall) and its irregular beadwork. I was intrigued by the way some of the circles didn't join up. It seemed to be mapping a territory I knew I did not understand, and therefore intrigued me more.

48 Beads and threads

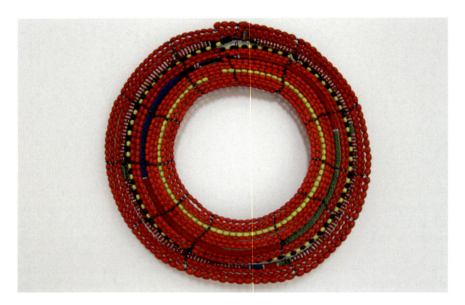

Figure 7.1 Maasai bead necklace.
Photo © the author.

Some years after receiving this present I went to Africa to make a film about literacy in remote areas of Kenya. For three weeks I travelled around with a local film crew visiting small villages and tribal areas. Here in makeshift classrooms built out of cement and corrugated iron, children and adults of all ages were being taught to read. This was a massive countrywide project, which was aiming to scoop up all those who had missed out on early schooling. It was a privileged way for me to see the country and to begin to understand a bit about the different tribal areas. In the north of the country we filmed the Samburu tribe, close relatives of the Maasai. The young men were learning to read and took time off from their cattle-herding duties to sit on hard wooden benches in the local classroom copying letters and words from a battered blackboard. The other groups of adults whom we had been filming were already quite integrated into the broad sweep of Kenyan culture. But with the Samburu it was clear that however advantageous being able to read might be for them, this marked the beginning of the end of their unique way of life.

At five in the morning we filmed the men and women getting up to let their cattle and goats out of the manyatta, the enclosure where they and the animals lived. We were all wrapped up against the cold and the young women emerged from their huts with red shawls over their shoulders caught up under piled-up cones of red beads. The light was just coming up and as the women herded the goats, the rising sun coated their necklaces with gold.

At the end of the filming I was invited to spend a few days with the cameraman and crew in a small camp on the border with Tanzania in Amboseli National Park. Here there were five tents on the edge of a small river, which we were warned hippos used at night. Giraffes stalked outside the tent area and the dusk was filled with unidentified animal noises. In the evenings we sat around an open fire, where we were fed steak and kidney pie and spotted dick straight out of an English public school. The camp cook had been taught his cooking years before by British settlers and was used to producing mounds of starchy food. Once dusk arrived and the fire was lit, young Maasai men, the *moran* from a local manyatta, drifted into our camp. They were adorned with deep scarlet red cloths, thin bead necklaces and sometimes a jumper or a woollen blanket – the drop in temperature in the evening was extreme. I was intrigued that they all wore wellingtons and was told this was a precaution against being bitten by snakes in the dark.

They came to sample our food, to talk and to check out the visitors. Having seen the Samburu women wearing necklaces much like mine I wanted to find out as much as I could from the Maasai and whether the colours and the way the beads were threaded had any meaning. One of the Maasai who spoke Swahili and some English explained that the beads were often organized in a way that showed the plan and shape of their enclosures – that they were in fact a kind of map. Maasai and Samburu manyattas are built in circles to provide the livestock and people with protection from marauding hyenas and big cats. The central hole of the collar represented the corral where the smaller vulnerable animals were kept. The alternating yellow and black beads around the edge of the collar mapped the fence, probably made of thorn bush, around the whole enclosure. The short lengths of beads delineated a family's huts, which might be arranged in terms of hierarchy. The different colours of the beads also had meanings. Red was for danger and bravery but most importantly it depicted the precious blood of the cows, which was an essential part of the Maasai diet. The green represented the grass, which came and went depending on the rain, and the blue beads were for the sky.

Hearing all this I realized that on my wall at home I had a highly personal account of a woman's place in her community and a map of where she lived. Other villagers would have been able to read this map and assess her position in her manyatta. I felt sad that I had this unique art work on my wall as it probably meant the woman was now dead, but I was also touched that the beauty I saw in the necklace now had a deeper meaning, which added immensely to my appreciation. Similar to a British landscape painting it depicted the land in which this unknown woman had lived, and like a watercolour of the chalk Downs by Ravilious, or a Turner painting of the Welsh hills, it was a territorial marker of place and identity. Something of this deeper meaning had conveyed itself to me when I hung it on my wall.

The following day we were invited by the *moran* to the manyatta. It was a settlement of about thirty-five people. The huts were tightly drawn together in rings around each other. Some of the women were wearing bead collars like mine, piled up in layers, others had many smaller beaded necklaces around their necks and heads. The more necklaces were worn, the higher the status of the wearer and the older the woman. Each woman had a different combination of beadwork. From a young age the women made their own necklaces. At various life stages a new necklace would be made. The beads were glass ones with an occasional plastic one breaking up the liquid flow.

The women walked us the mile to the stream where they collected their water and did their washing and then invited us into their tiny smoke-filled huts and showed off their children. The *moran* stood around watching this show of hospitality and then requested that we inspect their cows and goats. They were extremely polite and tried to contain their fascination with our bodies and our clothes. Anything of a bright colour was remarked upon, especially if it was red, and most of us, if the objects were the desired colour, gave away a belt or camera strap or woollen jumper. We (even the African crew who were based in Nairobi) were all similarly transfixed by them, by their lean muscular bodies, their red ochred hair and their perforated dangling earlobes. From a young age they had been trained to run fast and to hunt. They knew every hill and tree mass of their own land and those of adjoining tribes. The knowledge of their territory was in their bones and was an inherent part of their identity. There seemed to be a close link between land, manyattas, Maasai bodies and the beaded work that the women made.

On that day under a fierce sun my senses were assaulted by an overwhelming redness, the earth, the shawls and cloths and the ochre used as face paint as well as the blood of a slaughtered goat, collected in a tin bowl in our honour. Surrounded by the women with their collars of piled-up beads and enveloped with a pungent smell of cow dung, goats and sweat, I knew I would never look at my Maasai necklace in the same detached and sanitized European way again. What I didn't realize at the time was that we were filming a dying culture. The Maasai's rights to their land have since been steadily eroded and more and more of them have drifted into Nairobi and other cities looking for work. The women now make beaded necklaces on clean plastic threads for the tourists to take home with them. The link with identity and land has been severed and the beads you can now buy in Nairobi are simply examples of a craft. The art has disappeared along with the stories and myths it carried.

When I returned home I sniffed at my necklace hoping that, against all the odds, that pungent smell would have stuck to the beads. Sadly it smelt of nothing much, maybe just a hint of spray polish. However I still think of it as art, as it carries for me a potent sense of the culture it came from, the woman who made it and the connections it made for me with psyche. The art historian Michael Tucker makes a compelling case for viewing some contemporary art as infused with exactly these dreams and visions, which continue to connect with us in the same ways as so-called 'primitive art' has always done: 'the continuing mythopoeic significance of shamanic ideas of life can be detected within a great deal of the art of industrial culture' (Tucker, 1992: 50).

A few years later I travelled out to Bolivia with an all-female crew to make a film about women's groups who were organizing against government cuts and increasing poverty. Bolivian women had a history of being politically motivated and organized and this was to be one in a series of films to celebrate the UN Decade for Women, a hopeful and ambitious project to encourage women's equality worldwide. We filmed the Amas de la Casa in La Paz and the Women's Peasant Federation. During the time we were there a general strike was called to protest against the soaring inflation that was crippling the country. Acquiring enough cash for our daily needs was extremely problematic. When we went out to eat in the evening we had to carry a zipped-up bag full of paper money to pay for the meal. The money was counted out in the number of piles rather than individual notes, which by themselves were almost worthless. The country was in a desperate economic state.

I spent about a month in La Paz, first by myself setting up the contacts before the crew came out. I had a good translator and fixer who showed me around and fed me coca tea for altitude sickness. This helped with the blinding headaches and difficulty in breathing as La Paz is 11,913 feet above sea level. Walking around the city was exhausting because of the lack of oxygen and whilst I was there torrential storms washed rivers of mud down from the altiplano and through the poorer barrios, choking up the streets and making them impassable. Finding our way to the appropriate offices to gain filming permissions and the essential passes was a laborious task and I got to know the centre of the city quite well. On many of the side streets there were clothes shops that sold the traditional Bolivian skirts and bowler hats which the indigenous women wore. The many-layered skirts in multi-coloured fabrics hung in profusion next to thick piles of aguayos, the rectangular woven wool mantas and shawls worn by the Aymara and Quecha women. The colours of the chemical dyes seemed electric in the damp grey atmosphere. Pinks and blacks and vibrant greens shone through the mist, but there was something artificial about them.

In some of the streets though there were small stalls where women sold old aguayos, ones that had been dyed with natural dyes and woven from the wool of sheep or llamas. They were all unique in their patterning and colours and very beautiful. They reminded me of contemporary oil paintings – a block of brown or almost black thick but finely woven material would lie up against a thin band of cherry red. In another a zigzagging band of deep purple was woven next to a thin line of black and white interwoven wool. They were like canvases by the American painter Mark Rothko in their sensitivity to how one colour responds to another when it is placed next to it.

As I acclimatized and my headaches subsided I began to notice these older woven pieces across the backs of some of the women. Thrown across the shoulders they would then be knotted in front. Sometimes there would be a baby tucked inside, its presence only guessed at by a rounded form on the woman's back. Sometimes the aguayo was pulled round to the front to hold shopping or a larger child. These pieces seemed to be immensely strong and could deal with the cold and rain without the dyes running or the cloth shrinking. I became slightly obsessed with this art on display and would follow a good aguayo down the street, admiring it and hoping that the woman didn't become suspicious of my closeness. Unlike the modern equivalents, which all seemed to be of the same rather garish colours and patterns, every old piece was different, showing the weaving skills of the woman or, more likely, her mother or grandmother. The ones in La Paz had been made locally and seemed either to have geometric stripes of weaving running through them or a band with figures and animals. The first one I bought had dog-like creatures and birds with strange bent wings interspersed with flower shapes running across the middle of the dark brown wool. I was told the zoomorphic forms might represent the dreams of the weaver or be stylized animals important to the woman and her family (Figure 7.2).

I found this parade of creatures hypnotic and wished that I knew more about their origins. The red and green band would have been in the centre of the woman's back when she was carrying her child or just protecting herself from the weather. It was as if the woven animals provided a psychological protection as well as a physical one.

We spent two weeks filming our chosen groups of Quecha and Aymara women, who were using all the power they could muster to persuade the government to stabilize prices. The main focus was to force them to bring down the price of bread. In the bright cold air of the Andes we filmed an enormous rally of local women's groups displaying their union flags and banners. The men were relegated to the sidelines to watch as hundreds of indigenous women marched and sang their way across the altiplano. Each woman was wearing an aguayo, some of them made from the new chemical dyes but most had the muted colours of older pieces. As we filmed, a wonderful display of

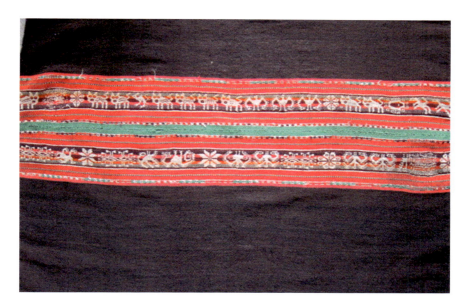

Figure 7.2 Bolivian aguayo.
Photo © the author.

indigenous art passed in front of us, the fine woven stripes of the cloths creating a haze of colour. They wound their way in a confident stream along the altiplano road showing off their solidarity and strength.

A few days later an enormous crowd collected in the central square in La Paz. The Plaza Murillo houses the Presidential Palace and the National Congress of Bolivia and had frequently been the battleground for resistance and power. Intense pressure was being put on the government to stabilize the currency. We filmed the gathering crowds and then joined the housewives' group, the Amas de la Casa, as they congregated in the square. Loitering men tried to prevent us filming the march and seemed disconcerted that we were women carrying film equipment. The local women understood this attitude well, dismissed the men, surrounded us and told us to follow them. They were used to demanding their rights, despite facing constant misogyny and extreme poverty. Most of them were carrying bundles on their backs wrapped around with aguayos. I felt as if the aguyagos were their battledress, their protection against the men and their jibes and against the dangerous political situation they were exposing themselves to and ultimately the harsh Andean weather.

Before we flew home I used any time I had to look for more aguayos. I was torn between the desire to buy the cloths and take them back to

London, and realizing that at some point it would be important for these antique works to stay in Bolivia. In the end I couldn't resist them and came back with five. I threaded the aguayos through loops and hung them on rods on the wall. For me there was no distinction between them and a so-called work of art, apart maybe from the original intention of the maker. My aguayos and my bead necklace have graced various flats and houses since then. They are undoubtedly women-made works, and they exhibit feminine strength and determination. They have deep stories threaded and woven into them and they are about belonging. But most important of all, as with all good art, they communicate these stories and the emotions of the makers.

Chapter 8

Struggle

In my forties I started seeing a psychotherapist. I had had an exhilarating time as a documentary film-maker. With the establishment of Channel Four and its broad-minded approach to film making I had been part of a group of film-makers whose ideas were encouraged, and I had flourished in a creative atmosphere and belief in the importance of using film to open up an understanding of the world. This period was relatively short-lived however as television was being deregulated and making films then had to take place in what soon became a bruising and underfunded marketplace. I realized that I would have to fight harder and harder for every film that I wanted to make and that compromise would be an everyday occurrence. I was also physically and psychologically exhausted from many years of trying and failing to have a child and I began to realize that my highly extroverted career in television was beginning to wear thin. I needed to change something and hoped that by talking to a therapist I might discover what that change might be.

My therapist was a Jungian and seemed inordinately interested in my dreams. Apart from the occasional nightmare, I had previously considered that my dreams were rather pedantic and dull and I had rarely remembered them. I started to keep a notebook by my bed and found I could remember more if I made a conscious effort on waking. As this process became habitual the dreams that I could recall increased, as did my interest in them. Occasionally the dreams were so full of intense images, physical sensations, feelings and even smells, that there was no problem remembering them hours and sometimes days afterwards.

A few months into this new process I had a dream unlike any other that I could remember, and it shook me awake. I realized with surprise that I was in the presence of the sculptor Jacob Epstein who wanted to show me his art. It seemed important to him that I responded to the dazzling array of his sculptures and drawings. At one point in this artistic immersion he opened up some heavy folding doors, on the inside of which were revealed shelves covered with artifacts, none of which, I was reliably informed by my dream voice, had been seen by anyone else before. There were small sculptures and pots and African figures. I could see every object in sharp focus and in the minutest detail, as if my vision had increased in acuity. I was aware in the dream that I was observing with extra sharpness and I woke up excited. My first thought was *how could I possibly have imagined or recalled these objects in such detail?*

I was not conscious at the time of having seen or of knowing much about Epstein, apart from his large public work for the TUC headquarters in London and his sculpture of St Michael and the Devil at Coventry Cathedral. I was amazed that I could have dreamt about an artist about whom I knew so little and in whom I was not consciously interested. My therapist gently suggested that this dream was about me, and about my need to open my eyes to something new. I was intrigued that I might unconsciously know more about Epstein than I was aware of. So, needing to find out what the artist might be able to reveal to me, and taking my therapist's interpretation rather concretely, I began to seek out his work. The timing of my dream was synchronous because the Tate had just purchased a major work by Epstein, which had apparently been looking for a permanent home for over fifty years. So I went to the gallery at Millbank to find out more.

Towering over visitors, *Jacob and the Angel* is a vast sculpture carved out of a single block of brown and cream alabaster (Figure 8.1). An angel with huge flat wings, like the open pages of a book, and sporting long flowing locks, bends his knees, the more easily to support the smaller figure of Jacob. The Angel's genitalia can be seen from behind where they have been forced backwards by the pressure of Jacob's body against him. The Angel's broad hands press into the small of Jacob's back pulling Jacob up and towards him as if in an embrace. Jacob's arms flop down over the Angel's biceps as if he is exhausted. He has his eyes closed and turns his face up towards the light whilst the Angel stares at Jacob directly in the face. He is so close that his aquiline nose is tucked in under Jacob's rounded upturned chin. Jacob could have fainted, or be asleep – the struggle is at an end. The broad relaxed face of Jacob is that of a child who has newly arrived in the world. His tight mop of hair is chiselled by small hard lines cut into the alabaster whilst the Angel's locks are voluptuous and smooth and show no signs of chisel marks. The Angel stands on his toes as he pulls Jacob towards him. Jacob's feet rest flat on the floor, but without tension as the Angel supports all his weight.

Epstein carved the alabaster so that the brown-red seams, which have vein-like marks running through them, make up the lower part of the two bodies, and the creamy part of the stone has been used for the upper bodies and faces of the two figures. It is as if the struggle between the figures has been so intense that all blood has drained away from their faces. The top half of the sculpture conveys a flesh-like delicacy whilst the torso and legs of the two men are full of blood, power and musculature. It is a monumental piece of work.

Struggle 57

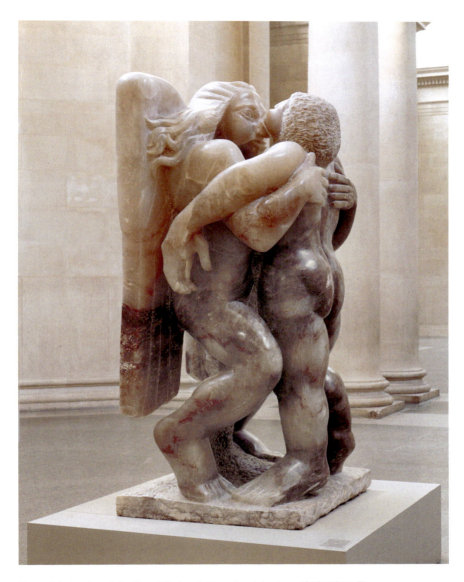

Figure 8.1 *Jacob and the Angel*, Sir Jacob Epstein, alabaster, 1940–1941. Tate. Photo © Tate.

I started walking around the sculpture to savour it from every angle, to see how the bodies pressed against each other and interlocked. I began to feel that I was looking at a most intimate creative act, not a sexual consummation, although the work is very erotic, but a fleeting moment of transition between one state and another that had been caught by the sculptor. A birth of a kind is happening as Jacob comes into being – he has been wrestling all night and by the light of the morning he has broken through into a different state. I felt the tenderness of the two figures, the sense of skin against skin and a childlike sense of being held by a parent, as well as the muscular power of the Angel and the exhaustion of Jacob. I badly wanted to touch the alabaster but resisted. I imagined that it was quite cool and very smooth to the touch. I felt tearful as if something about my own struggles had been acknowledged.

Despite its great size *Jacob and the Angel* made me feel that it was a private and personal piece of work, made because the artist had needed to make it for himself. It is of course based on the Old Testament story of Jacob who sends his two wives, servants and eleven children across the Jabbok river and is left all alone, whereupon he wrestles with an unknown assailant all night and does not give in. This figure wounds Jacob in his left thigh and in the morning, at the request of Jacob, blesses him because he has not given up the fight. At the end of the long dark struggle through the night and with the final coming of the dawn Jacob believes that it is God who has blessed him.

Epstein's sculpture does not feel like an illustration of the Bible story though, but rather that the artist had made an imaginative leap into the feeling elements of being alive in the world, and into the forces that as humans we wage against. Two male figures engage in face-to-face combat. One is smaller and less god-like than the other and yet does not give up. The sculpture conveys the exhaustion at the end of a struggle and the wrestling grip of the Angel appears to be more like a hug for the child-like figure of Jacob. Both figures have been changed by the encounter. It is a moment of deep connection; there is no longer any fight or need for competition.

The sculpture is about bodies; bodies that fight and bear down but also bodies that are capable of being very tender. In some ways it felt similar to Gaudier-Brzeska's drawings of wrestlers but on a much more personal and intimate level. Gaudier-Brzeska's wrestlers are synonymous with the collective as they represent all wrestlers. Epstein's figures are individuals. It felt to me that the sculptor was depicting himself in some kind of creative crisis and it left me painfully raw as well as uplifted. With my dream still very much in my mind, looking at *Jacob and the Angel* felt like an uncanny continuation of my sleeping state, as if Morpheus had had a hand in the carving of the work and then presented it to me in the Tate. It was early on in my understanding of dreams and I had yet to fully appreciate how they can reveal thoughts and images of which the waking mind is unaware.

Looking back now I can see that all that was necessary was for me to be visited by the artist in my dream, and then be prodded by my analyst to take the dream seriously. As a result, something had been woken up in me that had been asleep. I had become conscious of my present state of mind, which was both conflicted and exhausted. The sculpture was suggesting that struggles were not just necessary but worth it. The work had so impressed itself upon me that it was difficult to believe that I had not *found* it before. The more I discovered about the artist the more amazed I was that I could have connected in this way to a man who was as unlike me as I could have imagined. My therapist smiled when I suggested that I could see nothing of myself in Epstein.

Jacob Epstein was virile, combative and assured of his own qualities as an artist. He consistently attracted hostile and venomous attacks against his work and his own person. He was exactly the kind of acerbic and talented artist that the British found difficult to tolerate. He was born in 1881 in New York, a Jew with roots in Polish Russia. He left the States as a very young man for Paris and then London to get away from a family who were horrified that he wanted to be an artist. In the fifty-odd years that he worked as a sculptor in England he was never fully accepted until after his death. He was constantly attracting publicity around his uncompromising and very visible public works and his refusal to conform to Victorian expectations in his private life. The press attacked his sculpture as scandalous and inappropriate for early and mid-20th-century Britain and they pandered to a public who did not know how to respond to Epstein except with scorn and derision. He in no way fitted into society's ideas about what artists should create. The calm delights of the Bloomsbury Group and their decorative arts, or the sentimentality of 19th-century religious sculpture were in vogue rather than the large, brutish and irreligious works they saw coming out of Epstein's studio.

It is extraordinary to think that in the early 20th century the delights of Cezanne, Matisse and even Picasso were not widely appreciated. This was the conservative artistic background against which Epstein made his work, in a society that had yet to emerge from the Victorian era and saw the role of art to be soothing and reflective rather than to stimulate and challenge. Throughout the scorn and opprobrium that was heaped on him and despite the cancelling of his projects and the tortuous manoeuvres of the public departments which commissioned his work, Epstein fought on, refusing to be reduced by society to the confines of a respectable British sculptor, which he was not. He was supported at various times by other British artists, by a long list of benefactors and by his wives, his lovers and numerous children.

I soon saw that there was something very appealing to me about this non-conformity. This license to express oneself freely and be damned about what people might think had roots way back in my childhood, but had been encouraged by my love of both Matisse and Gaudier-Brzeska and was now fuelled by a large piece of alabaster in the Tate, which conveyed to me that personal struggle might bring release and new beginnings. I felt that I had been sad for too long about not being able to have children and had been filling my time up with work in an attempt to deal with these distressing feelings. Now I wanted to feel that there were positive sides to being childless, and that maybe after a period of what felt like stasis I could start growing again. I explored these thoughts in my therapy and realized that it might be time to give up the exhausting and extraverted immediacy of film-making and constant deadlines, and attend to my quieter introverted side, which might want something more reflective.

In my readings about Epstein I was surprised to discover that he had amassed a large collection of 'primitive' African and Pacific art. When I saw photos of these wooden sculptures I recognized them as the ones that had appeared in my dream. Epstein understood the power of these wooden sculptures and revered their simplicity of line.

> My African figures are wonderful ... they are genuine old works without a touch of European influence ... The effect can't be conveyed in words – to feel it they must be seen. The beauty of the lines, of the carving, the perfect realization of forms.
>
> (Rose, 2002: 80)

Epstein's love of what had originally been thought of by the British as ethnographic art, until he and other artists began collecting it, was driven by an appreciation of the aesthetic qualities of the works. He was sure that primitive sculptors were governed by the same traditions as modern ones and thought that the best pieces he had collected were made by highly individualized artists, and that rather than being primitive in any way, they were actually very sophisticated.

A few years later when I was working as a psychotherapist myself, I had a powerful experience in the presence of some Pacific art on a trip to Australia. Sheltering from torrential rain in Cairns in the Northern Territories, we had come across a warehouse full of wooden sculptures. Totem poles from Papua New Guinea stood beside piles of smaller sculptures from Africa and the Pacific. Birds with enormous beaks, masks with slits for eyes, black figures of Nigerian chiefs and carved twin doubles with blue bead necklaces stared at us out of the gloom of a grey Australian day. The smell of wood and feathers, of dust and trapped spirits was overpowering, the atmosphere heady with the whisperings of the dead. All these artifacts had been removed from their rightful homes and were now being displayed as works of art.

Despite feeling this dissonance I longed for my own wooden spirit from this highly charged atmosphere and I walked up and down between the piled-up sculptures waiting for one to call out to me. In the end I bought a standing figure of a man with his arms straight down by his sides (Figure 8.2).

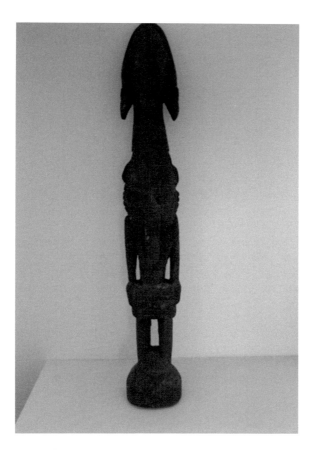

Figure 8.2 Papua New Guinea statue, wood.
Photo © the author.

He was about two feet high and had a flat elongated nose that turned under like a beak and rested on his chest. On the top of his pointed headpiece an animal, looking rather like a beaver, was draped head down, his forlorn face looking out at me. I was informed by the piece of scruffy paper nailed to the back that this figure from Papua New Guinea was used in houses to scare away the evil spirits. When I returned back home it became an important presence in my consulting room, calm, watchful and intriguing. In buying the man with the beaver hat I had wanted to take home with me a talisman of sorts, something to protect me and my patients from the sadness and anger that could be generated by the therapeutic work. It also seemed important at the time that my art from Papua brought something of *the other*, something of the collective unconscious into my London workplace.

I wasn't able to stay long in the warehouse. There was not nearly enough oxygen to contain all the emanations from these sacred wooden forms, each of them filling the space with their conflicting psychic contents and demanding their own place in the world. I needed air and went outside to breathe in the damp Australian mist. The dense accumulation of these sculptures had produced a perfect storm of psychic resonances, transferred from the societies and cultures where they had been made and now carried by these totemic objects.

When 'primitive' influences were seen to appear in Epstein's sculptures the conservative press railed against what they saw as his attack on British values. Rima, the heroine of Hudson's novel *Green Mansions* written in 1904, is a woodland creature half bird half human. Epstein's memorial to the writer is a stone relief depicting Rima surrounded by birds and foliage with her arms raised and open, almost as if she is supporting the weight of the stone above her. The *Morning Post* pronounced: '*Rima* is hideous, unnatural, un-English and essentially unhealthy'. The memorial to Hudson can still be seen in a quiet corner of Hyde Park, perfectly in tune with the surrounding trees. Rima's naked body is no longer a cause of concern and has long ago been cleaned of the green paint thrown at it in the 1920s.

Epstein was promiscuous and highly sexual but these energies were directly related to his desire for a child and his fascination with procreation. He was unable to have children with his first wife but eventually had five children from other relationships, two of the five children being brought up by his first wife. The years of infertility were extremely painful for him. Maybe they represented his own struggles as an artist at the time and his fears of not being creative enough. When he did eventually have children he was erratic in the time and love he gave them, and he treated his wives and lovers with variable amounts of attention.

His early distress about not making a child was carried through into some of his most moving work about conception and procreation. *Mating Doves* is one of these, a series of three sculptures expressing the stages of copulation, each one becoming more angular. This series of small sculptures explores the process by which two separate copulating bodies appear eventually to fuse into one.

The small delight of *Birth* (Figure 8.3) however, a stone relief carving of a baby pushing its way into the world through its mother's open legs, held the most engaging message for me. The birth appears to be happening upwards as the baby presses his tiny legs against the exit of the vagina, his genitalia hang downwards and with his bent arms he braces and pushes upward against this mother's thighs. His large head is raised, chin upwards towards the coming world. This is not a child moving downwards in the birth canal but upwards towards the light, the whole position, chin, arms

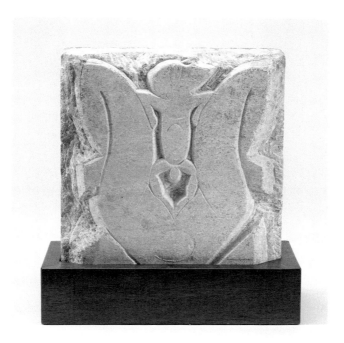

Figure 8.3 *Birth*, Sir Jacob Epstein, stone, 1913–1914. Art Gallery of Ontario. Photo © Art Gallery of Ontario.

and legs, mimics the position of the statue of Jacob, held like a newborn by the Angel, as if he too is being delivered into the world.

This baby is very active in his own birth. He is in the same physical position that Jacob is; head up, eyes closed, arms bent, legs loose, both of them exhausted but ready for a new beginning. For me, *Birth* linked directly to the idea that the birth of a child is simply the first of many births that may happen to this person, although, as I have argued elsewhere, these other births may be significantly different from procreation (Miller, 2008: 49).

This reverence that the artist conveyed in his work, for struggle and for breaking out/breaking through encouraged me to think that although I might not be able to produce a child out of my body, I could perhaps bring about other creative acts. It also helped me to change direction and begin the long training required to become a Jungian analyst.

Chapter 9

Multiple selves

I found my analytic training a demanding and a rather gruelling process, as it required me to hold two opposing positions simultaneously. The first was to be immersed in an ongoing analysis, which could reduce me to a childlike state as unconscious fears and anxieties from the past became more conscious. Here I was the patient. But in the second position I was learning how to be the analyst, which required me to think clearly and have intellectual rigour. When inhabiting this place I had to feel strong enough to see training patients and to try and keep, at least for some of the time, on top of the vast amounts of theory that had to be absorbed. It was the most demanding learning I have ever experienced, and far more intense than doing my university degree. I found it stimulating and fascinating but sometimes confusing as I switched between lying on a couch and talking to my analyst and sitting in a chair and listening to my training patients. Sometimes I was not sure who I was or which role I was fulfilling at any one time. This is a classic conundrum for all analytic trainees (Miller, 2000). I was often aware of experiencing myself as at least two, if not more, personalities – sometimes confident and in control, sometimes floundering around in a mass of feelings. Towards the end of the training when this duality had become especially acute, I found that I had an image in my mind of a painting that I had seen many years before in Mexico. It was not a painting that I had particularly liked at the time but it was now having resonances for me, which seemed important to pursue.

It was the 1980s and I was on a short contract advising a television company in Mexico about their programmes for children. A friend who was contracted to another television station travelled out with me. We stayed in a small flat in the centre of Mexico City and were driven to our respective TV stations early each morning. Although not far away, the journey could easily take two hours as the traffic crawled, hooted and juddered its way through the city. The congestion was chronic and the drivers were bad tempered, foul mouthed and exhausted. By the time we got to work the heat was intense, although it was still early in the morning, and I didn't relish facing an extended day with a very late lunch followed by evening work until 10 p.m., after which we ate. Late-night meals consisted of intense alcoholic drinks chased down with fiery colon-irritating food.

It was my first visit to Latin America and I was confounded by this topsy-turvy regime, which threw my body and mind into turmoil. I found the schedule very difficult to sustain and as the weeks wore on I got less and less sleep and ate very little. I was also anxious about the work and about communicating with colleagues in Spanish. My body was reacting to the extended day and, to add to the anxiety, we were often in minor car crashes and I frequently felt unsafe. Thankfully at weekends there were museums to be visited in the city. One day my friend and I braved the hot tarmac to go and look at one of the fresco cycles painted by Diego Rivera in the Ministry of Education. *Corrido of the Proletarian Revolution* is a monumental work depicting the Mexican people in domestic and battle scenes from the 1910 revolution. Here was something to which I felt I could relate. The boldly painted panels and bright colours reminded me partly of the rousing Communist posters that my father had brought back from Russia, and partly of paintings by the British painter Stanley Spencer, especially the ones depicting himself and his neighbours in the rural home counties in Cookham. This seemed like an oddly appropriate fusion of images to describe the Mexican Revolution – part glorious grand Communism, part small village community.

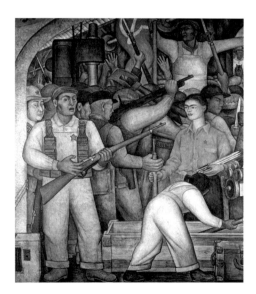

Figure 9.1 *Arsenal*, Diego Rivera, detail from the Ministry of Education frescoes 1923–1928, Mexico City. De Agostini Picture Library/M. Seemuller/Bridgeman Images.
© Banco de Mexico Diego Rivera Frida Kahlo Museum Trust, Mexico, DF/Dacs 2019.

In the centre of one of these panels the artist had painted a woman in an orange shirt with a red star on her chest handing out weapons to male revolutionaries (Figure 9.1). She had her black hair tied back, or maybe it was cut short; she could have been mistaken for a man. In her right hand she was holding a shotgun and delicately balanced in the crook of her left arm were long tubes of metal, which looked like paintbrushes but could have been rods for priming the rifles. This was my first introduction to Frida Kahlo, the androgynous revolutionary and the wife of Diego Rivera.

I was so intrigued by the figure of this female painter, whom Rivera had painted centrally in his panel, that I sought out some of her own paintings in the city. Kahlo was a prolific painter and her subject was almost always herself. Apart from a few luscious and erotic still lifes, all her paintings are self-portraits. The painting that I first saw in Mexico and that had come back to me so forcefully during my analytic training was *The Two Fridas*. Painted in 1939, it is one of Kahlo's largest paintings (Figure 9.2).

The two Fridas sit side by side on a long rush bench and hold hands. They are close and connected. Behind them thunderous clouds stream by, the weather is inclement. The Frida on the right of the painting is in traditional Tehuana dress, which she wore for much of her life. Her large red heart is outside her blouse with one artery wrapped around her arm. She is holding a miniature portrait of Diego Rivera in her hand. Another artery from the exposed heart wraps around the neck of the other Frida who is dressed in a colonial white lace dress with a flowered skirt. The colonial-dressed Frida's heart is also exposed through her torn dress and opened-up chest. An artery from this heart drips blood into her white lap while she attempts to stop the flow with a pair of forceps. When I first saw this painting I was both fascinated and repulsed. It felt like a painting full of pain, and it seemed like some terrible medical event had happened to these two women. With their hearts and their arteries exposed they were vulnerable to the tumultuous weather happening around them.

I remember looking at the painting and thinking that it was too graphic and disturbing to like, but that it was quite compelling. Both the Fridas seemed to be looking out at me with a combination of determination and sadness, a similar expression to those in many of Kahlo's other portraits. The fixed stare of the two women also conveyed a sense of secrecy; as if they knew something I didn't know, but had no intention of telling me. It was similar to that uncanny feeling that can be generated by meeting identical twins, when they appear to communicate in a private language with each other, but not to the outside world. The women's dislocation and pain was shown through their opened-up bodies and their clothes but not through their faces.

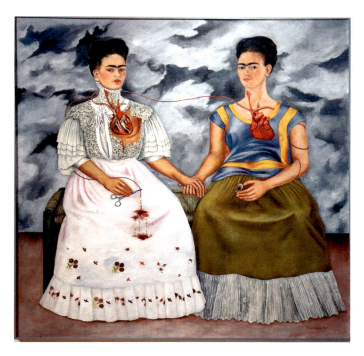

Figure 9.2 The Two Fridas, Frida Kahlo, 1939, Mexico City, Museum of Modern Art.
© Banco de Mexico Diego Rivera Frida Kahlo Museum Trust, Mexico, DF/DACS 2019.

The painting impressed itself upon me then as an attempt to present the dual nature of Mexican society through the two bodies of the painter. Kahlo seemed to be suggesting that there was an uncomfortable split between the indigenous nature of the people and the conquering colonial one. I understood the painting on this level at the time because of my own struggle with the exuberant yet death-loving Mexican characteristics that I was surrounded by. The indigenous and the colonial Spanish mix seemed to me to be an intemperate one, neither completely Indian nor completely European and resulting sometimes in death-defying behaviour. I saw the painting again many years later when it came to Tate Modern for a Kahlo retrospective, and then I could understand more about why it had resurfaced for me during my training, as an image of multiple selves that felt at odds with each other.

In *The Two Fridas* the artist presents herself as caught in the tension between the two cultures, but this tension is also a device to explore her recent broken relationship with Rivera; her two hearts are leaking blood. She has been wounded and a fracture of her self has happened. The two women hold each other's hand. They appear equal in this situation. Yet who is the 'real' Frida and can there be two of them? Which of them is most dominant? The effect of this doubling is one of extreme uneasiness. Uneasiness though is exactly what Kahlo wanted to convey. She painted this portrait after her divorce from Rivera and it underlines the broken heartedness of this event, although the two later remarried. It also suggests that it is the Frida in colonial dress who is more damaged by the experience and that the Frida in local costume is the one who still holds Rivera's portrait and whose heart is less damaged. My uneasiness with the painting felt similar to my uneasiness about my two simultaneous roles as patient and therapist that I was trying in some way to bring together. Was it possible to inhabit both these roles, or even just to inhabit the right one at the right time? Could one inform the other?

Kahlo was born in 1907, three years before the Mexican Revolution. Her Catholic mother had a Mexican/Spanish/Indian mother and a German father, so the artist's inheritance matched the mestizo culture of Mexico. She was in the perfect position to explore through her paint the boundaries between races, cultures and genders that was central to the Mexican psyche. In her self-portraits she exposed the deepest layers of her self and the many differing parts of this self. These layers cannot be seen in the depictions of her face though, which remain to a certain extent mask-like; her expressions do not reveal her feelings. The exploration takes place elsewhere, through the images and language of her paint, which questions neo-colonial cultural values, gender issues and female creativity.

Kahlo had debilitating polio in her youth, which left her with a limp. Then whilst still at school she suffered a major accident in a bus crash. She had originally wanted to be a doctor, but had to give up this desire after her accident. She spent the majority of her life in pain and strapped into a surgical corset. Rather than rejecting and abandoning her medical interest in bodies, she used the experience of her own maimed and transformed body as one of the major sources for her imagination. When she was in hospital after her accident she continued to paint whilst in bed. A mirror was hung above her so she was able to begin a process of intense study and replication of her own face. She also filled her house with mirrors. It was as if self-reflection became the modus vivendi for living. This modus vivendi then fuelled her quest for identity. Who was she really? She wasn't a mother and sometimes she wasn't a wife. Could she be a painter herself when she was living with a very powerful man who happened to be the most famous Mexican painter of the century? Her direct approach to these issues in her painting is why there have been so many feminist critiques of her work (Ankori, 2002).

She was also dealing with two life-altering traumas to her physical body. She had been cut off from her ability to have children and subsequently to walk without pain. After the polio at the age of eight she created an imaginary friend, quite a usual thing for a lonely child to do, but this friend could dance and move freely about and laughed a lot, unlike Frida herself. The friend became another Frida who was not damaged. Then, after the catastrophic bus accident that badly damaged her spine and her reproductive organs, she created the idea of the two Fridas in her mind. 'In the annuls (*sic*) of art, Frida is the only person ever to have ripped open her breast and torn out her heart to tell the truth in biological terms and say what it felt like inside' (Alcantara, 2011: 25). The artist shows us what the traumas she has undergone have done to her sense of self.

The defensive part of having another self touches on the psychoanalytic idea of splitting, the process by which a part of oneself that is difficult to face or is unwanted is projected into another person or part of oneself (Kalsched, 1996: 13). This splitting would have enabled her to stand apart from the damaged body, to be detached from it, in an attempt to distance herself from the pain; maybe the pain could be felt by the other Frida. The idea of having another self or a double, however, also enabled her to explore more deeply. If you possess another self or even selves, then that self can look back at you and describe what it sees as if it was another person. There can then be a conversation between the selves. I could identify with a similar need in myself, to inhabit the identity of the analyst rather than that of the patient when being the patient felt too difficult. But as the training progressed I became more aware of how essential it was to be able to inhabit both of these positions; that they were both going to be very much part of me and my new identity as an analyst.

Kahlo used her pain and her body in her art to constantly challenge the idea that she could be read as a single personality. She saw her identity as multifaceted and complicated. In *Self Portrait with Braid*, the artist presents herself as some kind of ancient goddess with her long hair knotted on top of her head like an elaborate crown. Exotic tropical foliage wraps around her, a tendril caressing her shoulder, as if she is born from the jungle. Around her neck she wears a heavy metal necklace with a small death mask attached. It is a compelling portrait of a woman identifying herself as carrying power, nature and death within her.

Kahlo explored these multiple identities at the same time as presenting a persona to the world as the ideal Mexican woman. The costume of the Tehuana woman which she adopted after marrying Rivera proclaimed her status as a traditional Mexican woman, a woman who is married and probably has children, a woman who wears her hair long and tied up on top of her head, a woman who has not adopted the dress of the conquering Spanish. It is this persona for which Kahlo is best known, her exotic highly decorated dress and her black voluptuous hair. This is the image that holds her together, both for herself and for those who look at her, and yet behind this image there are multitudes of other Fridas.

Kahlo showed me that her fractured self, which was so difficult for others to accept, held an important truth about identity. Our bodies are simply physical containers for what we like to believe is a constant state of being-ness. When that container is broken it is easier to see that there is no constant about it, we are all a multiplicity of ambivalent selves, moving and changing, and we cannot be reduced to a single identity (Kalsched, 1996: 113). My training as an analyst also showed me that there were many parts to the making up of myself and these parts were constantly changing in relation to each other. They might not sit easily together sometimes but they all deserved recognition, the child and the adult, the analyst and the patient, the introvert and the wild beast.

Chapter 10

Space

The summer after I completed my training as a Jungian analyst I attended my first professional international conference that was being held in Florence. It was August and stiflingly hot. The Florentines had long gone, leaving the sweltering city to the tourists and a few hundred Jungian analysts who were eager for enlightenment, friendship and the frisson of collegial disagreements. The conference took place in a modern building just outside the old town. Once inside the building I could have been anywhere in the world; utilitarian glass and marble, a vast semicircle conference hall and eyeball-drying air-conditioning were to be my environmental conditions for the next four days. Intrigued by the prospect of meeting colleagues from all over the world, I threw myself into the first day, attended the main events and smaller seminars and was excited to be surrounded by hundreds of other Jungian analysts. All the talk was about the fascinating psyche and how the unconscious worlds of patients, and analysts, reveal themselves through dreams, stories and images.

What I discovered though was that large groups of analysts in one place change the structure of the breathable air, which becomes weighted with unspoken meanings and interpretations. The knowledge that everyone there is interested, not only in the unconscious elements in their patients, but also in each other's unconscious depths, makes for an intense, close and sometimes edgy atmosphere. I had been through five years of training that had sensitized me to atmosphere, body language and all that is not said. In the room with a patient I had been taught to be open to both conscious and unconscious communications, but I had naïvely not anticipated that a large group of similarly sensitized people might generate an overload and bring about a short circuit in my nervous system.

By the second day, after a sleepless night in a tiny and airless hotel room, I felt disoriented and jaded. I wasn't sure how I fitted in with all these analysts and my habitual terror of being submerged within a large group came to the fore. I doubted whether I could survive the remaining days in these proscribed spaces. After breakfast, when I came out of the hotel, I longed to turn right into the old town where Florence was waiting to be explored, but instead I did what was expected of me and turned left, made my way across a busy main road and headed for the conference hall. Here, for the second day, in one of the most beautiful and artistic cities in the world, I inhabited a strange alternative reality of air-conditioned intensity. I attended talks, met colleagues and listened to papers delivered by Jungians from the USA, South America, Russia and Europe, who spoke of myths, beauty, disturbance and creativity. Many of the papers were fascinating, but I felt ill at ease. The multilayered city of Botticelli and Leonardo, of art and psyche, was breathing its hot breath outside the door, but I was cut off from it by steel and glass. I began to realize that words were not the way to connect me to the depths of the Renaissance psyche, and that I was being kept away from an experience I badly wanted; my body was twitching to come into contact with great art.

After another sleepless night I gave up any pretence of surviving the intensity of the conference and after breakfast turned the opposite way out of the hotel and towards the old town. I had been in the city a couple of times before but never by myself. Free to explore, I told myself that Florence was more important than listening to learned papers and I started to walk. Very soon I found myself in the square of San Marco, one side of which is taken up by the Dominican Priory, a beautiful building of pinkish stone with a church to one side and an internal courtyard surrounded by columns; a perfect place to stroll, rest and meditate. Inside the cloister the air was cool and there was space to breathe, the sounds of children, dogs and traffic abated. I felt weak with relief and exhaustion and sat down on a stone bench.

In the mid-15th century, a period we think of now as the early Renaissance, the Dominican brothers in Florence took over the Priory as their permanent home. Cosimo de Medici, the *de facto* ruler of the city and a supporter of the Dominicans, employed the architect Michelozzo to renovate the convent complex so that it suited the friars. Cosimo was a great supporter of their cause and paid the friars a weekly board. He also paid for oil, wood, salt, footwear and medicine and for the books needed by the friars for their study. This was to be a place where reading and contemplation could take place without concerns about bodily needs.

Guido di Piero, who took on the name Fra Angelico when he joined the order, had learnt to paint when he was a young man and on entering the friary he was asked to make frescoes for the communal areas and for all the monks' cells. The stated purpose of these paintings was to enable the friars to better understand the religious mysteries. The frescoes depicted scenes from the Bible, but were not simply narrative or decorative, as many frescoes in churches at the time would have been, but rather were to be used for individual meditation – mnemonic devices for the friars to use in their daily practice. These images were to be their companions on the road to a fuller understanding of the Christian faith. Unlike most religious paintings of the time, which were straightforward illustrations of the story of Christ, or were gilded and elaborated to suit wealthy benefactors, the frescoes at San Marco were made with a deeper purpose in mind, to enable connections to be made to a spiritual unconscious.

Fra Angelico understood that for his frescoes to work they had to encourage an imaginative space to be opened up within the friars' psyches, a space that engaged both the body and the soul and connected them to their own unconscious states. Each friar had a fresco in his cell, which he might live in for years. It was as if the fresco was an external projection onto the wall, of the friar's internal state. There he could see himself. As a result the frescoes became symbolic illustrations of the processes of the spiritual life and an external expression of a desired internal conversation. Fra Angelico was one of the first Renaissance painters to understand that painting had the ability to mediate conscious and unconscious elements in those who felt connected to them. This was partly an extension of the Renaissance idea that the individual rather than the collective was what was important and, as a result, personal experience was valued as well.

I knew none of this, almost miraculous, appreciation of what painting might do, as I relished the quiet of the cloisters and tried to clear my head of psychoanalytic theories of the mind. I looked for the entrance to the staircase that would take me out of the cloister and up into the north dormitory, the area where the friars and important male visitors used to sleep. The steps were very steep, requiring an effort to climb each one. I was soon pouring with sweat and I found that I was pressing my hands down on my thighs in an attempt to haul my body up to this private world of male religious practice. Before reaching the top of the steps I began to see the edge of a painted plinth with classical columns rising out of it and the dusty pink of a robe. On reaching the top I was gasping for breath and shaking with the effort but could now see that I was standing in front of *The Annunciation* by Fra Angelico; the first image to greet me and any other visitors who had climbed up to the north dormitory (Figure 10.1). As I recovered I thought of all those before me who had made this ascent and had arrived at the top in a similar panting state. I felt reduced to a frail body, only too aware of my physical limitations. But this loss of control over my body, which was now shaking, seemed to open me up to what was in front of me.

The fresco, the largest in the north corridor, was painted by Fra Angelico to encourage the friars and any visitor into internal reflection before reaching the cells. The perspective was painted to give the impression that you are looking through a window, beyond which is a loggia. Light is coming from the left as if from the garden or maybe it is coming from that real window in the north corridor? The Angel has come in from the garden and looks towards Mary who is seated on a simple wooden stool. Her blue cloak is wrapped around her legs and she has an expression of

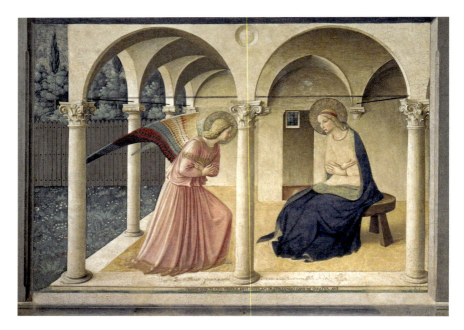

Figure 10.1 The Annunciation, Fra Angelico, fresco, c.1438–1445, Museo di San Marco, Florence, Italy.

Photo © Raffaello Bencini/Bridgeman Images.

concentrated acceptance on her face. Her hands are crossed on her chest. She leans slightly forward with her eyes on the pink-gowned angel who has appeared in front of her. Gabriel has long pointed wings, which reminded me of a dense multi-coloured woven carpet, and these wings are lit up from the light in the garden, or is it really that window in the corridor? Gabriel mirrors Mary's gesture with his hands. There is an empty space between the two figures as if there is a distance to be crossed between them; a void to be filled with their communications and this space is divided by a column that runs down the centre of the painting.

As my breathing slowed my eyes began to move between the two figures who appear so intently focussed on each other. Mary gazes at Gabriel with a calm, slightly sad acceptance. She has her hands crossed over her stomach, as if to say, *here, in my body, really?* Gabriel looks straight at Mary. Only his profile is visible, but there is a suggestion of a smile on his face. His hands are crossed over his chest and his knee is bent as if he is bowing towards her. He has just informed her of a fact that was unknown to her previously, and the two figures are lost in contemplation of each other and oblivious to my presence. I write 'oblivious to my presence', because my sense of looking in at a real event was so strong. A secret yet miraculous event was taking place in an ordinary setting – the Friary.

Fra Angelico had captured the sublime within the ordinary. It felt like the painter was able to see through the artifices of some of the Annunciations in churches and cathedrals to a profound human reality; that we have the ability to affect each other deeply through the words that are spoken and received. I was stunned by having this thought about a religious painting and wondered whether my insomnia of the previous nights was affecting my judgement. So I simply went on looking. As I gazed at the fresco I became more and more confident that I was looking at a work of art that had transcended the boundaries of its time and place and that by doing so it was saying something fundamental about the experience of being human. How do we communicate with each other? How does healing happen between two people? How is it that one person can effect change in another? What kinds of energies are generated by these exchanges? I felt that I was looking at a painting about what I might have been talking about at the conference, how two people really listen to each other and that, when they are able to do this, the space between them is filled with meanings and out of these meanings conceptions can happen.

The placing and situation of the fresco had helped me to experience this. The painting is part of the structure and memory of the building. There is no frame around it, apart from the painted suggestion of a window. Frescoes are intrinsically different from framed paintings in this respect, in that their boundaries leak onto the walls they are painted on. This lack of a frame encouraged me to believe that I was seeing something more like a scene from a dream or possibly even a hallucination, or a vision, either of which might be generated from inside myself. The lack of a boundary around the fresco put into question that it *was* a concrete external object, a painting; it could almost have been a projection onto the wall, of light and colour emanating from another place or another time.

Paintings that are inside frames signal to us that the inside is different from the real world outside. They suggest that it is safer to keep the imaginative space inside the frame separate from the outside, which belongs to another set of criteria. We are used to seeing paintings within frames and accepting this device. In front of *The Annunciation* I wasn't sure which world I was in. Was this Fra Angelico's creation or had he somehow managed to make me feel that it was my own imagined scene there on the wall?

Angelico encourages us to lose ourselves not just in this fresco and all the others in the friars' cells, but to use the building itself as an imaginative container, to experience the spaces of the Priory as places for the imagination to reside and flourish. In such spaces where the proportions, the architecture and the light enclose without constriction, at the same time as offering a stretching of the imaginative mind, creativity happens. It felt spiritual but not in a religious sense. I was being taken out of my immediate time and place and transported to a more diffuse area from where I could look at a part of myself in a fundamentally different way.

The achievements in perspective, which were brought about by the Renaissance, had challenged previous ideas about space and depth, but Angelico's art also questioned ideas about historical and personal time by suggesting that these might be less rigid than we like to think, and that art has the capacity to transcend these. He seemed to know that when art is placed in the right position in a building this can double the effect of recognition. It is then as if the art is entirely contemporary, there is no barrier of historic time to lessen the intensity of the effect. I recognized this timeless state as one I had experienced but not fully understood as a child when looking at a painting I loved. Now looking at *The Annunciation*, with past and present both stripped away, I was aware of inhabiting a more unconscious terrain.

It was as if I was being shown a world with fewer boundaries where new ideas might emerge. Distinctions between inner and outer, image and reality, were less clear. I felt that at moments the distinction between myself as a body and the painting as an object dissolved. This may be a similar feeling to those experienced by people who meditate frequently, a sudden letting go of the normal ties to the world. For five years I had been studying hard and immersing myself in psychoanalytic theories of the mind. I hadn't had a chance to see much art and therefore to remind myself of how important it was to me. Now, released from all the training, I could let go of the tension and it was as if I had suddenly been shown how these two interests might come together. How art and psychoanalysis might speak to and of each other. Here in the Priory the art had a very specific purpose that was not unlike the purpose of psychoanalysis, to enable a better understanding of oneself.

In the 1950s the psychoanalyst Marion Milner wrote *On Not Being Able to Paint*, a book about her difficult struggle to let go of her need to control herself when drawing or painting (Milner, 1957). When faced with a sheet of paper her conscious mind demanded that her hand should know at all times what it was doing and as a result her drawings were unimaginative and constrained. One of the conclusions she came to about these disappointing and very conscious creations was that painting and drawing had the ability to make new connections between the external world and her own internal responses to that world, and that she was unconsciously frightened of what these revelations might be, and so she held herself back.

Milner wrote that art could also challenge our profound belief that the boundaries between things in the external world were always secure and could therefore be relied on. This change of vision, which included the idea that boundaries might not be so rigid, might be welcomed sometimes, but mostly she found that she feared the idea. She observed herself as she drew, and she noticed that to allow her line to flow in her drawings and paintings, without trying to control it, meant that frightening images in the form of humans and animals appeared on her paper. Her unconscious mind had different ideas of what it wanted to express than her conscious one. As a result of her explorations she concluded that, 'painting is concerned with the feelings conveyed by space' (Milner, 1957: 12). I take this to mean that we are made anxious by the idea of open and un-demarcated space and that we prefer to know where we are. It is as if painting has the capacity to dissolve something that we thought of as intrinsically rigid and to remind us of these anxieties.

An unconscious aspect of being human is the knowledge (rarely acknowledged of course) that these so-called borders cross over and merge and interact in ways we would prefer not to know about. Art can stir up unconscious feelings in us, which we may try to resist. We may not want to know about our own hidden forces, which could up-end and challenge a more settled view of the world. It is a world partly known to us when we drink too much or take drugs. In these states the expectation is that we will return to a world of more fixed boundaries when we become sober. Although this merged world may be longed for as a world of no responsibility, it may also be resisted when we are sober as a place where meanings and identity can get lost. This place of lost identity is the place where artists create.

In my therapy practice I was getting used to the feeling of boundary markers disappearing when a patient and I were in a room together. Atmospheres, feelings and thoughts could travel between the two of us in often alarming ways. It was sometimes hard to know who was feeling what and whether the intensity of the atmosphere belonged to one person and was independent of the other, or whether it belonged to both of us. Untangling these affects is the stuff of analysis, but the way forward might be murky, dark and unsettling. If the feeling in the room wasn't coming from the patient then it belonged to me as the therapist, and I might not want to own that. Or maybe it belonged to both of us in different degrees and it had only become powerful because we had come together in this way. The process of beginning to unpick the genesis of thoughts and feelings and body responses showed how unstable and permeable these boundaries between us were. Sometimes we might be delighted by these contingencies but they might also appear to be worrying signs of a mutable world that scares us.

I can't say that I was less scared about the mutability of the world of the unconscious after my training and a long personal analysis, but I was more conscious of it and aware of its forces. In San Marco I began to appreciate how artists might be operating in some of the same in-between terrain as analysts, and that this was why I was attracted to both forms of human experience.

I lost my bearings in front of *The Annunciation* and when I returned to the building once more before going back to London, I lost my bearings again. It never occurred to me before going to San Marco that Fra

Angelico, the early Renaissance painter of such apparently simple and touching work, could have connected to me in this way. Whenever I think about *The Annunciation*, a postcard of which I keep in my study, I initially have the slightly vertiginous feeling of a door opening on a void; for a minute second there is a vast space, as if Angelico is asking a question I might not be able to answer, before the soft pinks and yellows and blues coalesce into the two figures facing each other across a loggia.

Chapter 11

The dream

As my interest in the world of the unconscious grew I was beginning to understand that looking at art did not always require a very conscious or a constant gaze; sometimes an inadvertent glance might be enough to hook me in. This had always been so of course, but I was now more aware of the power of the images, feelings and stories present in my unconscious world which seemed to have a magnetism all their own. When I found myself drawn to a painting almost without looking at it, it was as if the work was able to bypass this initial act of conscious gazing altogether and appeal directly to my unconscious. Works that did this seemed to enter me through my eyes but then veer off on a different path and I would then respond to them from my gut.

One of the reproductions hanging in my parental home had been *The Snake Charmer* by Henri Rousseau (Figure 11.1). The inky black figure of the naked woman with yellow eyes and playing a pipe had fascinated and frightened me as a child; whilst the twisting black serpents reaching out of the forest beside her haunted my fantasies and my dreams.

Because I saw the painting every day it became familiar but it was also an unknown; a mysterious image which never seemed to give up all its secrets. Who was the naked woman with her long black hair falling down her back and what was she doing standing on the edge of a lake in the moonlight? Why were the snakes and the pale pink spoonbill so entranced by this silent music?

I got to know Rousseau's other jungle pictures through reproductions and loved them for their dense flat colours, their odd animals and their strange plants. As a child I felt that there must be stories behind all these paintings. They had an illustrative quality that appealed to me and I found the imagined jungles exotic and compelling, even though some of the plants seemed to be suspiciously like the rather ordinary European plants that my mother grew in pots at home. Despite these anomalies the green density of the jungles and their capacity to be the shelter for a multitude of animals infected my young imagination. Later, when I started travelling and saw some tropical forests for myself, I was surprised and slightly

80   The dream

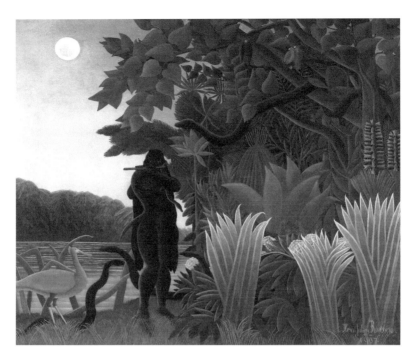

Figure 11.1 The Snake Charmer, Henri Rousseau, oil on canvas, 1907.
© Musée d'Orsay, Paris, France/Bridgeman Images.

disappointed by their airy sandy greyness and lack of green density. These thinner wispy jungles seemed to lack depth and stories.

As I grew up I was delighted with Rousseau's childlike landscapes of Paris, his portraits of oddly shaped people and children with their totemic cats and puppets. But despite these passing delights, I continued to think of him mostly as an artist who had delighted me in my childhood because of his jungles. It was not until a major exhibition of Rousseau in London in 2005 that I saw and was subsequently enchanted by *The Sleeping Gypsy* (Figure 11.2).

The Sleeping Gypsy painted in 1897 is one of Rousseau's largest paintings and, unlike the more congested jungle pictures, it is full of sky and air and space. Against a vast starry firmament a lion, with a perplexed expression, peers down at a sleeping gypsy. The gypsy, unaware of the large beast beside him, sleeps deeply, his mandolin at his side. He holds a staff in one hand and his other arm is bent back supporting his head. He is wearing a robe of many colours and lies on a striped blanket. His water pot stands

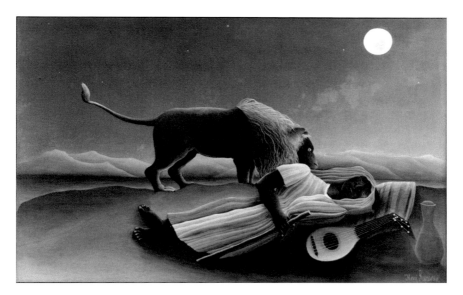

Figure 11.2 The Sleeping Gypsy, Henri Rousseau, 1897.
Photo © Luisa Ricciarini/Bridgeman Images.

sentinel beside him. A white full moon casts a narrow shadow on this scene but the light comes mostly from the front, from the viewer's perspective, flattening the image against the background. As in most of Rousseau's paintings, there is very little attempt at perspective.

My first response to this painting was sheer delight, as if the painter had opened up a door for me to see into another world, which was at the same time both familiar and strange. Human and animal were placed here together in an odd juxtaposition, which could be either peaceful or menacing; there seemed no way of knowing. The landscape was more like a moonscape than a desert, and through this moon-desert flowed a blue/grey river bordered by pale pink hills. The gypsy's possessions looked like paper cutouts stuck onto the canvas, almost as if they had found their way there from another painting. Yet despite these oddities it did not jar in any way. Although strange it also appeared true, and seemed linked to a core of certainty deep inside me. *This is how things are* I thought.

My body responded unconsciously to this painting as if it was communicating a profound truth about the world and about how we experience it, in the same way that a dream might do. I surprised myself, and the woman standing next to me, by emitting a sigh as if of recognition. This was the first time I had been so aware that the world of the unconscious *was* the world that Rousseau was attending to in his paintings. This idea did not appear to sit easily with most of the critiques that I had read, which labelled him as a naïve painter and therefore rather superficial.

Rousseau was born three years after Renoir and four years before Gauguin in the small town of Laval, into a petit bourgeois family. He spent the second half of his life as a painter in Montparnasse alongside the Impressionists and Post-Impressionists and later also Picasso, who respected his work. Initially he worked as a customs officer, a douanier, a collector of tolls, and gave up this work in midlife to concentrate on painting. The fact most frequently cited about Rousseau is that he was self-taught and did not take lessons to learn to draw, which was then a requisite for all artists of the period, whether they were able to show their paintings at the Academie des Beaux-Arts or not. He longed to be accepted by the Society des Artistes and by the establishment, although this was never likely to happen, as he was criticized for his lack of training, his apparent inability to master perspective and his unrealistic juxtaposition of natural elements. He produced work unlike any of his contemporaries' work, which seemed untouched by either Impressionism or by his times. French society's view of Rousseau was that of an innocent, someone who was always outside the establishment. They saw him as fitting into no school except his own. These sentiments added weight to the idea that he could be dismissed as a naïve artist who had not learnt his trade.

Some of his fellow artists thought differently though and appreciated that Rousseau was a painter who was able to paint from deep inside himself and to produce canvases that were radically other. Picasso, who bought some of Rousseau's work, immediately recognized him as a great artist. 'The first work by Le Douanier that I had occasion to buy grew inside me with an obsessive power … It is one of the most truthful French psychological portraits', he said of *Portrait of a Woman* (Morris & Green, 2006: 175).

Picasso also organized a party in honour of Rousseau to which artists, poets, critics and dealers were invited. Some of the guests treated this occasion with gentle mockery but the poet Apollinaire wrote a poem in his honour and became one of his main champions. Rousseau's supporters appreciated that the painter was doing something which none of them could do and that to dismiss him as untrained was to miss the point. They understood that the painter was looking inside himself for inspiration rather than out at the world. This difference in perspective enabled him to do his work without being particularly affected by other painters. All around him the Impressionists were blurring the line and dissolving shape in their attempts to paint the effects of light. For Rousseau line was pre-eminent and the refraction of light of little interest to him. His gaze was fixed on archetypal images from his internal world. He wished to reveal the magical and collective aspects behind our accepted sense of reality.

Looking at *The Sleeping Gypsy* put me directly into a dreamlike place. I found myself staring at different points on the canvas and losing myself in a meditative state. The water pot is a pot from another age, an archetypal image of an ancient pot; a pot that I recognized and felt I had seen many times before. The mandolin is a mandolin that has been played over centuries, an object that has both a past and a future life, and seems to miraculously appear again as the same mandolin in some of Braque's paintings, such as *Still Life with Mandolin*. The gypsy with eyes closed but lips open recalls African sculptures made out of a piece of hard, black ironwood. The lion with his magnificent mane, tucked in like a rug under the fold of skin at the back of his neck, is a beast of fairy tales and legends who might have appeared in *The Just So Stories* by Kipling and who certainly reappears as Aslan, the all-seeing and all powerful lion in *The Lion, The Witch and the Wardrobe* by C.S. Lewis.

The lion's tail, with the beautiful hairy brush, holds him in balance against the night sky. Everything is absolutely still. The lion and gypsy are not breathing, the water in the river does not run. The whole is immobilized in its archaic yet perfect structure and all appears totemic. 'A great work of art is like a dream; for all its apparent obviousness it does not explain itself and is always ambiguous' (Jung, 1971, para: 161). This is a painting that convinces, not because of its reality, that can be seen and reproduced on canvas, but because of its dreamed reality, another kind of reality altogether which we can learn to understand and which may mean something to us. A dream has its own coherence and its own logic. Jung, in one of his most important insights, understood that this dreamed reality used a different language: 'It (the unconscious) develops motifs that appear across time and across cultures in myths and fairy tales in similar forms. These same primordial images pervade our dreams, fantasies and ideas even today' (Jung, 1984).

When I first started analysis, I found it difficult to engage with my dreams as they seemed so ordinary. I was only walking to the bus, or meeting my brother, or worrying (still, as an adult!) about doing an exam, I would say dismissively to my analyst. My dreams all seemed to be about nothing very much or certainly about nothing important. The objects and people I had dreamed about were known to me and therefore not surprising, or they were not connected to strong or memorable feelings. But when I was encouraged to tell the dream as best I could, something different happened in the speaking. The known objects and people often came together in an altogether different conjunction from the one that my conscious mind wished to relate. They then seemed to have been put together by my dreaming mind to form an image or story or a feeling that when examined resonated as something other. The images remained familiar but the feelings associated with them felt like they came from a deeper place.

This resonating *something* might bring with it surprise or longing or resistance and then be recognized as meaningful with another part of my understanding. Dreaming of doing an exam might suddenly link to another pressure or requirement in my life that was making me feel the same as when I was a child. This ability of the dreaming mind to make meaning out of known or found objects or events is a sort of *bricolage* of the unconscious, where chaotic events and objects are brought together. The images that the dreaming mind uses are not just those consciously known to us, but they also come from the collective unconscious, an unconscious world of images that is shared by us all. This storehouse of images is something that Rousseau intuitively understood and explored.

The French writer Yann Le Pichon researched the original sources of Rousseau's images and discovered them as found objects. He tells how as a child he was taken to visit Rousseau's sole surviving child, Julia, and she gave him an old album to look at called *Betes Sauvages*, which was published by the Galleries-Lafayette department store. It contained 'two hundred amusing illustrations of the life of wild animals with instructive texts'. He identified a photograph of spoonbills that looked as if it had come straight out of *The Snake Charmer*. He checked this immediately with a reproduction of the same painting that was hanging in Julia's room. 'This bird with a long, flat bill struck me as resembling the one on the edge of the moonlit lagoon, enchanted by the naked Negress who is intent on charming entranced pythons with her flute' (Le Pichon, 1985: 21). Le Pichon then went on to discover photographed and drawn sources for many of Rousseau's pictures. They were easy to identify because in many cases the painter had reproduced the exact position and expression of the animal. The lived reality was not what was important to him, it was the archetypal elements that Rousseau was searching for.

Since then other researchers have tracked down many sources of drawings, photographs, stuffed animals and animal sculptures which the artist used as direct references for many of his pictures. There is a stuffed animal display of a Senegal lion devouring an antelope which was made for the 1889 opening of the Zoological Galleries in Paris that has been copied exactly by Rousseau for his painting *The Hungry Lion*, which he painted in 1905. A lion could be copied just as well from a taxidermy display in the Jardin des Plants or a picture book. For his purposes he did not need to draw animals from life. All these models and illustrations served the same purpose; they were to be plucked from wherever they were available as useful representations of *the* lion or *the* monkey or *the* exotic plant of our unconscious dreaming life. As well as frequenting the Jardin des Plantes for images of animals and examples of vegetation, Rousseau also went there to get himself into a certain state of mind: 'When I enter those hothouses and see those strange plants from exotic countries, I seem to fall into a dream' (Morris & Green, 2006: 41). The presence of the exotic, the other, induced in him a hypnotic state, which he was then able to translate into painting.

He also went for walks in the countryside outside Paris and brought back armfuls of leaves and flowers, which he drew faithfully, regardless of whether the flowers or foliage were appropriate for a tropical forest environment. They were simply tools to help him to represent the world of his imagination, which then connected him to deep layers of his unconscious. He would make sketches in the countryside and then return to his studio to create a painting. During this process he then appeared to disregard his initial realistic three-dimensional drawings and reduce his knowledge to strong outlines and flat colours. It is as if he was affirming that this was not a plant that exists externally in the world, but rather one that resides internally in the depth of his and our psyches. However, to discover this internal image he had to start with the external reality, the accepted view of a plant, and then make the journey inwards to that other imagined plant that we all somehow recognize.

When I was looking at *The Sleeping Gypsy* it was as if the mandolin and the water pot and the lion and the moon had been through the same kind of metamorphosis. They were still recognizable as the objects and the animal that they were but they had lost their individuality and taken on a universal quality.

The Sleeping Gypsy is a painting about our shared world of myth and archetypal images. Part of the allure of the painting for me, and what adds to my fascination, is that it presents a subjective as well as an objective position. The gypsy is both the dreamer of the painting of himself, the lion, the night sky and the unmoving river, at the same time as being the subject of the scene. He is both the dreamer and the dreamt. When looking at the picture I could experience the scene as if it was inside the gypsy's mind, as well as at the same time recognizing it as part of a collective experience of all those who look at the painting. These two positions add to its mystery as a painting of the conscious and the unconscious simultaneously. Rousseau shows that these two states are inextricably related.

Rousseau, like all Parisians, lived in a society that was becoming immersed in new ideas about the psychological forces that control us. In 1889, twelve years after he had painted *The Sleeping Gypsy*, the first International Congress of Physiological Psychology took place in Paris. The idea that there was an unconscious state in all of us was becoming more widely accepted. Picasso could see that his fellow artist's paintings were psychologically acute despite the apparent simplicity of his images. The painter was exploring the idea that there were primordial images accessible to us all, which could put the psyche into a state of enchantment and which had certainly affected me as a child and then again as an adult.

By 1912 Jung was identifying these images as promoted by what he began to call the collective unconscious. These images, he suggested, were similar everywhere, their main features being that they were unconscious but that they always carried a charge, a numinosum. 'The *numinosum* is either a quality belonging to a visible object or the influence of an invisible presence that causes a peculiar alteration of consciousness' (Jung, 1970: 6). We might experience this kind of numinous moment when we see something that we believe we have seen or even heard before, although on a conscious level we know that we have not. Or an image may have the effect of jolting our conscious mind to a realization on a deeper level, as if connected to a different level of energy, or a sense of the spiritual. This alteration of consciousness by exposure to the jungle, the exotic, the other, was what Rousseau experienced in his visits to the Jardin des Plants, and which he then conveyed through his painting. To be able to use images of animals and people and turn them into hypnotic pictures, he would have had to put aside a large part of his ego as a painter and allow himself to be influenced by the images coming up from his psyche. This would be similar to him being in a dream state, where consciousness falls away leaving him exposed to a highly active unconscious state.

On a conscious level Rousseau was in control when painting. He apparently could see the entire picture in his mind before he began and would draw it all out on his canvas and then meticulously paint it in from the images in his head. But he then became so receptive to how these images from his unconscious affected him that he sometimes terrified himself and had to open the windows in his studio to let in fresh air and let the terrors out. This apocryphal story about his fear of his own creations has sometimes been presented to support the idea that the painter was simply naïve; that he must be so if he could be frightened by his own block-like and unrealistic animals. Like Matisse, however, he knew that the act of painting was not a benign act, but one that stirred up the unconscious mind. The animals on the canvas were directly related to those beasts we are aware of being in touch with when they surface in our dreams. They may not look like the lion or tiger we know from the zoo, but they are potent dreamed animals that carry with them a host of associated feelings. They have not been filtered through a conscious thinking state or returned to the realistic forms of a rational thinking mind. The lion in *The Sleeping Gypsy* is no longer a lion from a photograph or a lion shut in a cage in the Jardin des Plantes, it is a beast of terror and power but also warmth and tenderness. It is the lion inside us all.

Rousseau worked within an area of enchantment, a potentially dangerous space, where representing unconscious processes might become a volatile task. He understood that painting could, in the right circumstances, cross over a boundary and link us to a dimly seen yet mostly unknown world, a place where images spontaneously appeared that we had no control over. It was as if Rousseau was able to plunge head first into that unknown world, the world that I had become more aware of in front of *The Annunciation*. This was the place where boundaries between the conscious and the unconscious are more liquid than we imagine or wish them to be. Picasso, who was delighted by Rousseau's work, understood what an alchemical and magical process painting could be. In a conversation with Francoise Gilot he said: 'It (painting) isn't an aesthetic process, it's a form of magic interposed between the hostile universe and ourselves, a way of grasping power, by imposing a shape on both our terrors and our desires' (Rousseau, 2006: 198).

Art has the capacity to show us that the boundaries between our conscious and unconscious worlds are areas of slippage and seepage rather than areas of rigid demarcations. The act of making art not only reveals this slippage but attempts to fix it in the form of painted images and, as Picasso suggests, by shaping 'our terrors and our desires' it gives us an illusion of control over the unknown-ness of the unconscious parts of our natures.

Chapter 12

Silence

The experience of unknown-ness in art was to follow me abroad. On a brief holiday in Germany away from my therapy work, I stayed in Dresden to meet friends, experience the rebuilt city and to look at the art. Dresden is a Baroque city that has risen phoenix-like out of the ashes of the firebombing rained on it by the British in 1945. The major buildings have been reconstructed stone by stone, partly from those original blocks that could be recovered and partly from newly hewn ones, all in an attempt to heal the catastrophic wave of destruction that once blew them apart.

The Rococo city hugs a bend in the river Elbe, again showing off its grandeur and prestige. The skyline of the river frontage is a cacophony of statues, globes and gold leaf, rebuilt to replicate the previous glory that was Dresden. The effect is dramatic but rather unsettling. The checker-board effect of the old blackened stone and the newly quarried creamy yellow blocks is a constant reminder of the city's devastated history, but this mixture of old and new feels unstable, as if the city might yet again break up. To be in Dresden is to feel that one is being constantly questioned about the past for it is a city of unquiet memories.

Dresden is also one of those European cities lucky enough to house two paintings by Vermeer, that quintessential painter of the Dutch Golden Age who is known mostly for pictures of quiet contained bourgeois interiors; delicate paintings of 17th-century rooms of apparent peace and quiet. We made our way along the grand riverfront to The Old Masters Gallery, one of the vast rebuilt buildings. It is dark and lugubrious and houses an extensive collection of painters from the 15th to the 18th century, all of which were hidden in a safe place during the war and have now been returned to their rebuilt former home. I was looking forward to a respite from the sense of unstable uncertainty from the rebuilt city. The rooms in the gallery are tall and echoing, the violent magenta-papered walls fight with layer upon layer of pictures, jostling each other for space. Initially it was difficult to take in the extraordinary range of artists housed there, and I found myself dutifully checking out the Raphaels, Titians, Rembrandts and Rubens with interest but a certain amount of emotional detachment. There was far too much to take in. So I passed by these great masters and went in search of two of Vermeer's earliest paintings, both of which threw me into more uncertainty and an unexpected and acute state of unknowing.

The earliest of the Vermeer paintings in The Old Masters Gallery, *The Procuress*, was painted in 1656 and is one of his largest paintings (Figure 12.1).

I was at first very surprised that it was a Vermeer, because of the size, the style and the subject matter, none of which fitted with my preconditions about the painter. The painting depicts the buying of a young woman for sex. Four figures lean into the picture and over a beautiful oriental carpet. The young woman who is being procured is modestly dressed in a white cap and a brilliant yellow jacket. The man paying for her favours leans over her, coin in hand ready to drop it into her outstretched palm, whilst his left hand rests on her breast. Despite the apparent coarseness of this transaction there is a gentleness and intimacy between the two figures who have agreed the deal. The couple are bathed in light, a light which separates them slightly from the procuress herself, an androgynous figure

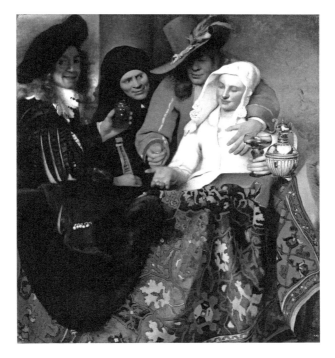

Figure 12.1 The Procuress, Jan Vermeer, oil on canvas, 1656. Gemaeldegalerie Alte Meister, Dresden, Germany.

© Staatliche Kunstammlungen Dresden/Bridgeman Images.

in black with a slightly menacing smile who peers round at them from the back of the painting. A man on the left of the picture in a large black hat looks out at us, smiling. He is not part of the threesome but rather a voyeur of the scene which is unfolding before him and us. Some scholars believe that this onlooker is a self-portrait of Vermeer, which suggests that the painter himself is implicated in the looking. We are implicated too in the looking, the sexual unease and in the strange unsure relatedness between the four figures.

The paint is applied more thickly and roughly than in Vermeer's later smaller paintings and it felt to me like he had not yet refined his style, or maybe it suited the slightly coarse subject matter. This is one of the few paintings known to exist of the artist's attempts at subjects of Bordeeltje or low life. In the mid-17th century when he painted *The Procuress* there was a flourishing group of Bordeeltje painters who painted brothels and street life, often lascivious in content. Yet this painting is not really comparable with those other painters of the period. Vermeer's involvement in his subject matter is completely different from the illustrative and voyeuristic approach of painters such as Van Baburen for instance who made no social comment on the scenes of lascivious men and prostitutes that he was depicting.

Vermeer's prostitute has a mind and body all her own. The expression on the face of the young woman is of fondness towards her customer and certainly not one of guile or submission. The couple seems to inhabit an erotic closed world, set apart from the greedy eyes of the procuress and the voyeuristic ones of the man in the hat. I felt drawn into the scene by this couple, as they appear untouched by the dark figures around them. It is as if they share an understanding that protects them against the monetary transaction of which they are a part. They exude a powerful interior quality of mind, as they are absorbed in themselves and their own thinking. This self-absorption separates them from the two dark figures, as well as from myself, the beholder of the painting. The luminous young woman in yellow with her pink cheeks and downward contented gaze reduces the other figures to minor characters in the story. She seems to be lit from within by her ease and enjoyment of her own body and the erotic transaction of which she is a part. She is not a victim, and she rejects the idea of herself as an erotic object. She does not allow us to think of herself like that. As the painting slowly affected me I realized that I did not see myself as a voyeur of this scene either, but rather as an amazed onlooker who had been allowed to experience this young woman's sense of power.

I found myself asking questions about this painting like: 'What was this young woman really feeling?' 'Does she agree to this transaction?' and 'Isn't the couple too tender for this to be about an exchange of money?' These are not the kinds of questions I would normally be interested in asking about a painting, but Vermeer had hooked me into a questioning space that enticed and irritated me and defied expectations. Although initially frustrating, this void eventually grew into a creative place from which I could properly look at the work and ask a rather different question, which was, 'why was Vermeer confusing me?' The confusion seemed to be about an initial mismatch between what I expected of the painting and how it actually was.

To appreciate how it actually was appeared to depend on my ability to give something back; not to interpret but to become involved in a part of the artist's thought processes and to see where that took me. Vermeer seemed to be more interested in painting the calm interiority of the young woman than fulfilling any expectations I might have had about the subject matter. It was as if, whilst painting, he was acutely aware of my physical presence looking on. Almost as if the most important thing the painting could do was to encourage an internal dialogue in myself, by being silent and not answering the questions it posed. I felt I was being encouraged to participate in the young woman's experience without being able to ask her the questions I wanted to ask. Vermeer was in love with his depiction of the girl, with his own desire to show her as a person who lived in that moment, a person who was truly alive.

This experience of questioning followed by introspection on my part seemed to parallel a process that I might experience in my consulting room. Facing a patient who I was finding confusing I would ask exactly the same kind of questions of myself. 'Why is this patient confusing me? What does she need me to be drawn into? What part of her inner world does she need me to see?' I would use myself as a sounding board to try to understand what I was being told. I was familiar with this process of interaction but never in quite this way when standing in front of a painting.

I knew from previous Vermeers that I had seen that the painter was a master of the mysterious. Silence emanates from his paintings. Art critics vie with each other to produce new interpretations of why the painter has such a hold on a 21st-century audience. Mostly these interpretations circle around what hidden truths can be revealed to the uninitiated, and how objects in the paintings, such as bowls of fruit or musical instruments or open doors, are symbols redolent with back-stories, which may offer us the promise of a finality of a story. This interpretation of symbolic objects is an attempt to control and understand the painter's imagination. What I had not really grasped until I saw *The Procuress* was that Vermeer is a painter who *wanted* to put me into a state of un-knowing. This state was inevitably frustrating but I began to glimpse that it might also be a highly creative act, one which threw me back on myself; to use myself to find my way.

Many Dutch painters of the period made their living painting such scenes of bordellos, yet Vermeer didn't stick with this subject matter and, within a year of painting *The Procuress*, he had produced his first quiet painting of an interior with a figure, *Girl Reading a Letter by an Open Window* (Figure 12.2). For the remainder of his life he painted what we

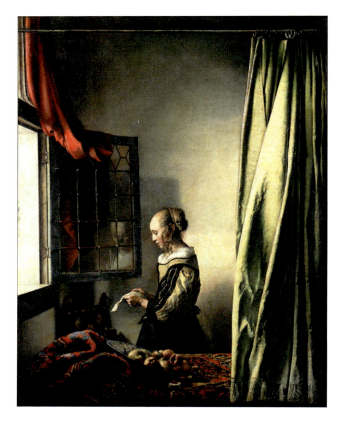

Figure 12.2 Girl Reading a Letter by an Open Window, Jan Vermeer, oil on canvas. Gemaeldegalerie Alte Meister, Dresden, Germany.
© Staatliche Kunstammlungen Dresden/Bridgeman.

now think of as typical Vermeers, studies in calm domesticity, paintings which appear to show intense psychological insight. It is as if the painter's initial interest in the external world of religion, power, money and sexual favours had swung dramatically to the other end of the spectrum, into a smaller internal world of thoughts and feelings where the room depicted becomes part of the subject's and the beholder's imagination. Or had he always been interested in his female subjects' internal worlds? Maybe the trajectory was more of an obvious one, the beginning of the artist's quest to engage the beholder in a fascinating communication with female interiority in painting?

Girl Reading a Letter by an Open Window is the other Vermeer owned by The Old Masters Gallery in Dresden. It is a small, intense painting of a young woman standing by the light of an open window reading a letter. She is in profile but I could see a faint reflection of her face in the glass. The picture is swathed in fabric. A red curtain is draped over the window and a luscious rug is bunched on a table in the foreground. Drawn back like a stage curtain there is a heavy green silk drape framing the scene, encouraging me to believe that I had been allowed to gaze for a second on a private moment, a moment of concentration and reflection. The letter has the woman's full attention. It is half read, as the upper half of the letter bends back tantalizingly over her hands.

I wanted to know what was in the letter and whom it was from. I was lucky enough to have been shown something that would normally have been private and yet I had not been given the full story and, insatiably curious, I craved answers.

This canvas has been X-rayed as many of the Vermeer canvases have, in an attempt to delve deeper into the mysteries of this enigmatic painter. We know from the X-rays that Vermeer had originally painted a picture of Cupid hanging on the wall behind the young woman and above her head, but that he then removed this and in its place a tall blank plaster wall remains. The picture of Cupid would have been seen at the time as a direct reflection of the content of the letter; that it was a love letter, but Vermeer has decided not to allow us this information and so without it we are left to speculate about what kind of a letter it is that the young woman is reading. It is as if the X-rays simply throw up further questions. A scientific approach will never provide the answers to uncovering the painting's meanings.

After some time in front of the painting I was able to let go of a desire to find a narrative. I then began to notice something far more interesting; that I was experiencing a state of mind that was present in another person. I did not fully understand the state of mind of the young woman or appreciate its subtleties, but Vermeer had made me believe that what was important in my looking was to notice her moment of aliveness. If this young woman knew that I was looking she would not have been so entirely in her own time and moment and unaware of her physicality. By seeing her I was able to recognize those moments in myself, when I lose awareness of my body and my surroundings for brief periods of time. This unselfconsciousness and emotional intensity in the painted figure was the same as I experienced emanating from the young woman in *The Procuress*. The painting of the young woman reading her letter exuded psychic concentration. She is unaware of her physical self, the external world is, for a moment, lost to her and so it was on some level to me. I knew that it was a delightful room with a scarlet red curtain draped over the window and a beautiful oriental rug covering a table, but these visual elements seemed to be part of the emotional state I was experiencing rather than just objects in the room.

The room had an organized balance with a purpose to it. The placing of the curtains, rug, bowl of fruit and bare wall all helped to focus my attention on the light coming in from the window that was falling on the young woman's face and her letter. All these props expressed an aesthetic that delights in everyday things and in their capacity to carry atmosphere.

Vermeer used corners of his house and his curtains and rugs as movable props. The same carpets and chairs and windows appear in many of the paintings in different positions and for different effect. The painter was eliciting an emotional response in me by apparently painting reality. As the writer Rebecca Solnit wrote: 'It (Art) makes mute objects speak, and it renews the elements of the world through the unexpected, or it situates the everyday in a way that makes us wake up and notice' (Solnit, 2013: 193).

This lovely room drew me into a well-organized bourgeois household, where all is domestic calm. But once in the room I discovered that what was important was the body of the young woman and the intensity of what she is experiencing, or what I imagined she was experiencing. Vermeer is an enormously seductive painter. He fills his paintings with his own intense loves and desires and then dares us to step inside, with the suggestion that we might have our own desires fulfilled. Once seduced he keeps us looking and questioning.

Sitting with not knowing is what we have to do with this painting. If I had not been reminded of sitting in silence with a patient this process might have angered or annoyed me because of its refusal to answer my questions. Vermeer's stillness and silence could be seen as an aggressive act against the beholder's own stream of thought. His stillness questions our own un-stillness. His silence attacks our own constant need for answers. We are the fidgeting, hopping, demanding and un-relaxed figures in front of his canvases. This painting, as well as being about the experience of silence, is also about the power that the young woman holds, because she is the only one who possesses knowledge of her inner life.

The art historian Bryan Wolf suggests that this attempt to convey silence does have a historical and social context, in that the upper bourgeoisie, of whom Vermeer was a part, experienced 'privacy and inwardness as signs of leisure that distinguished it from other social groups. The goal was to render private what before had been part of a public set of codes' (Wolf, 2001: 158). Being private cuts us off from others. It suggests that the other person or social group is not needed. If Vermeer was painting a class signifier, he also cleverly uses this to cut us off from a full interpretation of his paintings and to make us work.

Being frustrated in this way did not initially appeal to me and I wanted to resort to the easiest explanation, whether the picture actually gave this to me or not, so that I could feel more in control and less ostracized. However, staying with this feeling that I could never fully know this painting and the tantalizing aspects of that eventually offered me something else. If Vermeer is suggesting that this young woman has an inner world that will always remain unavailable to me, this is a truth about all of us, whether or not we want to accept it; there is always a distance between ourselves and others that is full of un-knowing.

What then fascinated me was that Vermeer understood that wanting to know what we cannot know is a psychologically acute way of getting us to really *look*. There has not been an artist since Vermeer who has managed to engage the viewer in quite this specific way. He transfixes us, not just with his painterly brilliance but also by stimulating our desires to enter into the world he has created, he demands our concentration and our imagination and poses questions that he does not answer.

This approach speaks very powerfully to me as a therapist because one of the most difficult crafts to learn is to be able to sit with a patient and bear the not knowing, to wait and see what happens. Sitting with not knowing is the centre of the creative work and out of this state can come new knowledge, which could never have been imagined or thought about before. Bearing the unknown reminds me that there will always be far more about this person that I do not know, than the stories, characteristics and emotions that I do, and that to jump to conclusions will close the work down rather than open it up. In these kinds of situations in the consulting room I would allow my fantasies and images a free rein and then notice what came up. This free-floating attention is the same as that which I was made to bring to *Girl Reading a Letter by an Open Window*. Sitting with un-knowing is of course also associated with religious or spiritual states of mind, and Vermeer's paintings have the ability to put me into a space that can feel spiritual. 'What matters in painting is *pushing* the mundane toward the instant of transcendence', writes the art historian James Elkins (Elkins, 1999: 188).

Girl Reading a Letter by an Open Window is of course an object, but it is an object that is not simply a thing. The painting radiates a capacity to engage the beholder in an act of self-exploration. It is a painting that has its own emotional life and its own reality beyond the painter and the paint, and thereby can retain its secrets and its own mystery. It has transcended its physical state as an object and become more real than reality, which always has transience built into it. The mystery about the painting is an intense one and it is in this place of mystery where the sacred and the human come together. Or, as the writer Siri Hustvedt suggests about another Vermeer painting of a young woman, '*Woman with a Pearl Necklace* was something other than what it appeared *to* be' (Hustvedt, 2005: 12).

Vermeer has the extraordinary capacity to make a work of art that is not just suggestive or emblematic of another life, but that is able to live independently, a work that exists separate from the painter and then affects the beholder as if it has come into being all on its own. Looking at these two paintings in Dresden reminded me of the process of sitting with my patients. Both patient and painting are alive and have rich internal worlds.

Chapter 13

Alchemy

The frame around the painting, which looks as if it might have been gold, has been stippled over with black or maybe dark blue paint, in an attempt to break up its antique nature and straight lines. Some of the stippling crosses the edge of the frame onto the painting itself. On the left of the picture three upright blocks of dark colour lean precariously against each other pressing against the edges of the frame. On the right is another brown block separated from the three on the left and apparently being pushed towards the right by a green form stippled with red blotches and in the form of an enormous K. The bottom edge of the K is painted over the frame at the bottom. The form on the right stands against, or is it *in* an orange field covered with small green dots? Above the large K there is a purple square sitting on a background of dull yellow and the same black stippling as on the frame.

'What does it mean?' asked the woman standing next to me in front of this painting by Howard Hodgkin entitled *Dinner at Smith Square*. 'I simply don't understand it' (Figure 13.1). It was 2006 and we were at a Tate retrospective of Hodgkin's work. I made a garbled attempt to put something of what I understood of the painter into words. 'He paints experiences and the feelings about those experiences. The titles give a clue as to what the painting is about, but they don't necessarily help.' The woman remained confused. 'I can't see anything in this picture that relates to a dinner.'

> That's maybe because what he is painting is his feeling reaction to a memory of this situation. He's not painting the dinner with people eating but rather a memory of what the experience made him feel like. I suppose that initially what we can get from it is that it was rather dark and sombre and that there were layers of feelings on top of each other connected to the people present and almost obscuring each other. Maybe there was someone rather forceful there who is represented by the brown pillar on the right. It is a painting about one dinner, one event which made an impression on him. And if we look and wait feelings may also be evoked in us by the colours and forms.

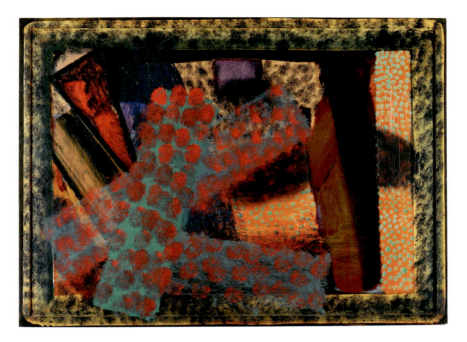

Figure 13.1 Howard Hodgkin, *Dinner at Smith Square*, 1975–1979, oil on wood.
© The Estate of Howard Hodgkin.

She thanked me unconvinced and moved away.

I had no idea really what I was talking about either, as using words to explore a Hodgkin painting is not always helpful and made me feel my attempts were clunky and ridiculous alongside the physical and emotional sensations elicited by this painter's work. I have found when looking at Hodgkin's paintings that these sensations can be powerful and intimate but extremely difficult to hang on to. When they come it is as if there is an electric charge between the painting and myself. It is recognition of a shared but partly unconscious feeling state. It seems to me that when this happens Hodgkin has touched the deep core of what paint can do, that it can sometimes have the ability to transcend its thing-ness and inhabit another realm where it becomes the direct carrier and conveyor of feelings.

That art can use space to recall and reignite memory is a theme of many of the artists in this book but for Hodgkin it is the core of his work. Many artists transform space into compressed memory and this is part of the task for Hodgkin. He painted, not just to record a memory, but did this also through eliciting the feelings from that time, so that they can then be experienced in the here and now. As the artist Celia Paul says: 'Painting is the language of loss' (Paul, 2019: 152).

I had gone to this exhibition worrying about a patient I was seeing at the time. He was feeling very angry and I was concerned that he might act on his destructive feelings and harm himself. I hoped that I had put everything in place to give him enough to hang on to and to choose life. I had not consciously thought that looking at Hodgkin's work might help my anxiety or my ability to help my patient, but as I spent longer and longer in front of each painting I began to feel lighter. It was as if the intensity of the experience of living that Hodgkin managed to convey counteracted my own feelings of doom. It wasn't simply that his paintings expressed happiness, some were concerned with states of depression and sadness, but they felt truthful and they explored our ability as humans to feel a wide variety of emotions. They also reminded me that this is what life is, a series of feeling states. I wondered whether, when I returned to my consulting room, I would be able to convey to my patient Hodgkin's ability to pin down and honour tiny moments in time, whether they were difficult or celebratory ones, in a way which might be helpful for this man; that all feelings are transient eventually.

Clean Sheets is a smallish, oblong and very green painting (Figure 13.2). A thick circular brush mark of rough acrid green covers over the frame and within this are blocks of darker green and black/green paint. In the

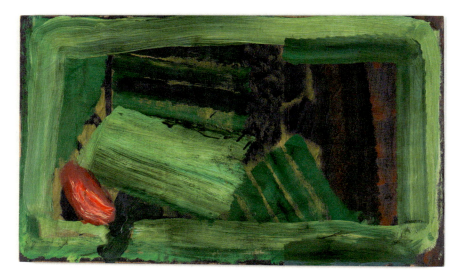

Figure 13.2 Howard Hodgkin, *Clean Sheets*, 1982–1984, oil on wood.
© The Estate of Howard Hodgkin. Photo © Tate.

bottom left corner a curve of red/pink paint suggests a body, but only one body. This is a shut off space, nothing and no one can enter. This is a cold clean and lonely bed and feels to me like a painting about desolation. By first remembering and then painting and communicating this feeling Hodgkin contains it; something I hoped my patient would be able to do.

Hodgkin is different from all the other artists in this book in that he painted his experiences and therefore potentially also our experiences of what it feels like to be alive at any moment in time. Other painters can sometimes elicit this feeling in me, they can stun or surprise me into living in the moment but they do not describe the actual experience in paint as Hodgkin does. Hodgkin was an admirer of Matisse and, like Matisse, he had a belief in the capacity of paint to carry and convey strong emotions. Both artists painted interior and intimate situations where peculiar emphasis may be placed on specific things that are then somehow weighted with significance. Matisse painted the objects and people that obsessed him, a jar, a plant, an open window, a model in striped trousers, all conveying an importance and intensity of mood. Hodgkin carried this intimacy one step further. His life's work was about how to explore memory, and how to notice how some things or events are remembered with much more significance than others, especially those that evoked strong emotions. It was in the painting of these moments of reality, which coalesce around feelings, that Hodgkin believed he could communicate with the world at large.

This kind of sensitivity in an artist requires a responding sensitivity on the part of the viewer and a willingness to look and wait. My response may not be similar to that painted by Hodgkin, but his truthfulness then elicits a feeling that *is* truthful to me. I have some sense of conflicted feelings between people in *Dinner at Smith Square*, but I may not have read this in the way that Hodgkin painted it. However my reaction is still valid because an object that I have been staring at has elicited an affective response in me, which I find meaningful.

Contact with a painting by Hodgkin can sometimes feel to me fleeting and difficult to hang on to. For a second, a memory or feeling of my own may be physically present, brought about by colour, form or an over-layering of paint. This instant, though, is like a transitory glimpse of gold. It is there and then it has gone, but I have experienced it and feel the richer for it. For this reason admirers of Hodgkin's paintings can feel enormously grateful to him for this gift. 'They (the paintings) require that their vulnerability be met and answered by an equivalent vulnerability on the part of whoever engages with them' (Graham-Dixon, 1994: 40). The painter's generosity is well known and this comes from an intense desire to communicate: 'Obviously my "language of forms" has far more than a physical purpose. Alone in my studio, working on my pictures I long to share my feelings' (Auping, 1995: 79). This intense desire to communicate his feelings is at the centre of the artist's work.

I had seen small exhibitions of Hodgkin's work before the Tate exhibition, but it was this retrospective that showed me the consistency of his ideas about painting and how unique and revolutionary they are. Each white-walled room was carefully and sparsely hung so that the pictures did not fight or infect each other. His paintings seem to leak colour and emotions, as if once they had reached the stage of conveying what has been aimed at they cannot fully be contained or controlled; they acquire liquidity and movement. It is not just the blazes of luminous paint that need to be given room, but also the intensity of contemplation required by the viewer if one is to make a connection with the painter's mind. A bit like wine-tasting, the process of looking at Hodgkin's paintings demands clean air and a clean palette in the form of an expanse of white wall before moving on to the next painting, each one requiring eyes and an imagination that is newly washed.

This is totally unlike most of my experiences of looking at lots of pictures in galleries. A recent exhibition of garden pictures, *Painting the Modern Garden, Monet to Matisse*, was closely hung together and exhausted me because of a surfeit of both good and bad paintings. They did not encroach on their respective spaces, contained within their often elaborate frames they behaved like paintings who knew their place, to delight, maybe even to excite, but not to ask for or give more than that. As a result, the space between the pictures was immaterial. They held themselves in check. Hodgkin's paintings do not hold themselves in check.

It was at this Hodgkin exhibition that I had recognized that I had a recurring physical symptom when looking round exhibitions. Often my hearing would become blurred and sounds become distant as if my ears were blocked. I suddenly understood that this strange symptom of *exhibition hearing loss* actually helped me to see. I was not distracted by sounds in the gallery or the people around me, and this heightened my ability to look. When I came out of galleries my hearing always returned. This response of my body to looking at pictures was confusing until I realized how helpful it was when looking at Hodgkin's work. It was a protection against erroneous stimulation, because one of the thrilling things about looking at his paintings is the sense of imminent danger in being a beholder. Hodgkin's art works do not necessarily know their place. They have the ability to transmit their power across a gallery towards anyone who is receptive. Once caught by their beams I have no control over my responses and am surprised into states of mind I had long forgotten about. His paintings are charismatic and invade like an electric shock, as if a boundary has been broken open between the external thing, the painting, and my internal world – a breach has been made in the dam. Colours clash and slide towards each other in vertiginous waves. My vision is directed towards this painted thing, yet my mind is turned inwards as if paint had transmogrified before my eyes and changed from being a concrete viscous colour into a light that is reflecting my internal feeling state. At this retrospective exhibition I felt that the alchemical process of turning matter into spirit was right there in front of me.

Like the alchemists, Hodgkin worked at turning paint, the base material, into gold. We may think of the 12th-century alchemists now with understandable scepticism, as a group of men who, through their material and spiritual quest, believed they could discover the centre of all things by turning *base* materials such as iron and lead into *noble* ones. 'Alchemy first of all is a master of perversion' (Elkins, 1999: 149).

> Alchemical metamorphosis is not so much pre-scientific as parascientific: it works alongside science (from para- meaning 'beside') by taking some laws from the rational world of experimental procedure, and fusing them to irrational methods designed to expose the unpredictable properties of half-known substances.
>
> (Elkins, 1999: 122)

This struggle to turn the matter of the world into valuable and highly prized commodities, which carry spiritual meaning, has some affinities with the ways in which Hodgkin talks about the painting process. 'For me I have often said, the subject and object must become one thing. If this doesn't happen then for me there is nothing – the picture doesn't exist' (Auping, 1995: 69).

Jung became interested in alchemy because he saw it as a metaphor for understanding the symbolic nature of the unconscious. He thought of it as a historical precursor to a modern study of the unconscious. The painter David Parker explores the relationship between painting and alchemy:

> both painting and alchemy appear to create a unique and special bond between material substances and psychological processes. Without such a bond, it is probable that neither painting nor alchemy would hold such intense meaning and fascination for their practitioners.
>
> (Parker, 2008: 45)

In the 1970s Hodgkin was thrilled to discover a new material substance that enabled him to paint over his oil paint far sooner than the usual days or even weeks required for drying time. This speeded up his painting process, maybe allowing it to be more in tune with his thinking and feeling processes. Liquin is a fast-drying alkyd medium that increases the flow of oil paint and intensifies its translucency so that previous layers show through more clearly. In *Clean Sheets* I could see through the top colours to the layers of paint underneath. It is as if the artist's memories are built up of accretions of images and emotions, layer upon layer.

One of the paintings I was most affected by in the Tate retrospective was called *Bombay Sunset* (Figure 13.3). The picture shouted its sunset moment to

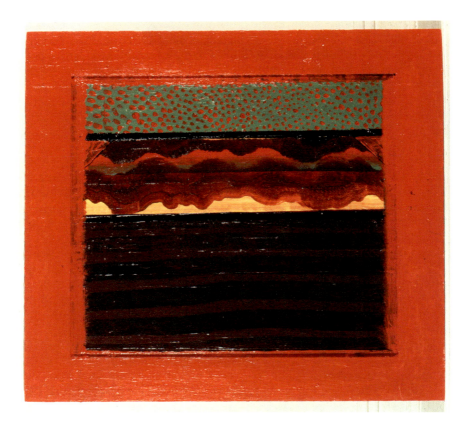

Figure 13.3 Howard Hodgkin, *Bombay Sunset*, 1972–1973, oil on wood.
© The Estate of Howard Hodgkin.

me across the gallery. Superficially it appears to be a representational painting. It is almost square. It has a wide frame painted thickly with orange/red paint, the same evocative deep red for me of Matisse's *Red Studio*. In the foreground, and taking up half the picture, is a field of brown horizontal stripes. Where this ends an orange sky is visible beneath red clouds, which drop from another horizontal line above which the red-tipped clouds rise up towards a brown sky, which is again interrupted by a black line. In the corners, made by the black line and the frame, two triangles of wood have been inserted and painted red. It is as if the painter wants our eyes to be forced further into the depths behind. Above the black line small stippled red dots appear over an emerald green background. The red paint spreads from the frame onto the painting, as if the painter has carelessly missed the edges. As described,

Bombay Sunset can be imagined as simply a succession of horizontal lines and blocks of colour above each other, yet this is a painting of enormous depth.

I dislike most sunset paintings and often find actual sunsets ludicrously sentimental, as if the wonder of living on a planet in a solar system had lost all meaning and been highjacked by photography and the world's easy emotions. *Bombay Sunset* erased that in an instant and showed me what charge a sunset can carry. Maybe that is because the painting is not simply a representational one. I can read it as a sunset but it is primarily a painting about feelings, and it is because of the feelings that the picture evokes such power. It seems to me to be about Hodgkin's response to being in India. It is as if he has spread out his soul on the land of India and it has met him with equal intensity.

Hodgkin first visited India in 1964 and became enamoured of the country: 'the moods, the way people live in India that has probably influenced my painting very much ... very much. It's the sort of nakedness of their usually very inhibited emotions. I mean everything is very visible, somehow there' (Serota, 2006: 176). What the artist seems to be suggesting is that, despite a personal reticence on the part of Indians, the experience of the land and its people generate a multiplicity of emotional states that transmit themselves to him. These are feelings that in our cold, reserved Northern climes are more difficult to access or have different colour resonances. *Bombay Sunset* conveys a heat beyond anything we might experience in the West; it is fiery and dangerous and inhospitable to man, yet thankfully the tumultuous raging sun is dropping behind the horizon and soon the land will feel cooler.

On my first visit to India I was astounded by the sun's capacity to boil and spill its burning air onto the land and people. On a trip I made before the advent of safe bottled water, I dehydrated quickly and my legs and ankles swelled up. I thought my brain was being slowly but surely fried and I had to resort to lying in the shade for hours with my legs up against a tree. Sunset was a blessed relief for the land, the people and the animals. Having always loved the heat, on this trip to India I longed for the evenings. This was a time for moving about again, for eating and relaxing. In India I began to understand the point of sunsets; they were a dramatic marker of a change in the day, a chance to recover and renew physical capacities.

Bombay Sunset reminds me of that intensity of light and heat and the sun's struggle to keep up its broiling, even as it slips behind the edge of the earth. The painting is a memory of one such evening when it seems the heat will never abate and the land will never cool. Colour becomes broken up and separates from its moorings as if it is no longer contained by objects but becomes free-floating blobs and lines. The over-heated air moves in waves as if it too is melting. The painter shows this alchemical effect as red dots on a green background and a bending and curling of light. It is disturbing to mind and body and can generate hallucinatory states. I remember a few occasions when, lying supine on a hard bed, soaked with my sweat, I felt that if the sun didn't go down soon it would be me who disappeared over the edge of the world first. This experience of dissolution by heat would never be an experience that could be had in Britain, even in very hot summers. It was this stark difference, and the sense of otherness, that made me love India and crave her extremities, her craziness, her colours and her beauty when I was not there. *Bombay Sunset* is about a burning out-of-control madness, as far away as possible from the muted colours of England and the reticence of most English painting.

Hodgkin is a well-known collector of Indian art. I saw some of his collection when they were on display at the Ashmolean in Oxford and hankered after many of the pictures. Most critics have presumed that Hodgkin's collection of Indian paintings has a direct relationship to his own work; that they reflect the colour and vibrancy of India, the India of our imagination and the India of miniatures. However his collection of pictures does not contain many miniatures and they are often not highly coloured. Many are from the Kota School, low-toned relatively large paintings and drawings. They do not seem connected to the painter's own ecstatically vibrant palette, nor are they typically religious paintings, which many of the Indian miniatures in collections in this country are. They are carefully collected depictions of domestic scenes, animals and social occasions.

Andrew Graham-Dixon, in his book on the artist, argues convincingly that one of the appeals to Hodgkin of these works is the depiction of shared experiences between people, and that the Indian artists' ability to convey a world of interiority also relies, like Hodgkin does, on a variety of painted codes – flat patterns for decorated cloths, simplified linear lines for an elephant in movement and very realistic painting of a character's flesh. All these methods are used together to create a unique world (Graham-Dixon, 1994: 118).

Indian art does not adhere to rules, it simply does what works best to create a specific feeling or effect, just like Hodgkin's art does. 'In Indian painting I have found much that for me could be found nowhere else, but I cannot tell you what – I can only metaphorically wave my arms at the pictures – and say look!' (Hodgkin, 1991). This made me think that what Hodgkin loved about India and some of its art was that, from a Western perspective, it is primarily about difference, about a spiritual way of being in the world, which is quite alien to many Europeans' sensibilities, but has strong affinities to Hodgkin's own paintings.

Hodgkin was an obsessive worker but, like all obsessives, he was searching for an alternative level of being. His art uses and transforms objects in the external world to focus on the internal. So a painting may appear to show what something looks like, but it is actually really a painting of what that thing or incident felt like to the artist. This transformation of an object or a person or situation into the feelings they generate was a Herculean task and paintings took him years to complete. He used to place his work in progress with their picture faces against the walls of his studio, until he was ready to turn one around and contemplate it. He then spent a long time looking and waiting until a colour or brush movement seemed appropriate. Painting over and layering or pentimento was a large part of the process. We can often see through the most recent brushstrokes to those that lie beneath. Many things are partly hidden and may only be experienced as a shadow of an idea or a feeling that lies somewhere between a conscious and unconscious state.

Hodgkin always worked on a fine edge with very little room for manoeuvrability. At any moment he might fall into confusion on one side or over-explicitness on the other. It is this awareness of danger and the bravery with which he faced his task that I admire so much. To paint what it feels like to be open to the loves and oppressions of others, their vagaries and their delights, one cannot have a hard carapace; in fact it is better if one has fewer layers of skin. But this is an anxious and vulnerable place to be and Hodgkin was an anxious painter. He was consistently exposing himself to his internal world and to the landscape of emotion that he found there. One situation may have impressed itself on him as worthy of revisiting, a dinner party, a moment with a lover, or how another person affected him. He then might have spent years on a painting, leaving it and revisiting it constantly until the shapes and the paint formed a memory image.

Hodgkin always experimented with borders and frames as if he was aware that where the paint meets the world is the place at which it is most vulnerable – where the delicacy and slipperiness of the emotional state can be most infected or affected by brushing up against the other – that is not of itself. The edge, the transition, is what he protects his paintings against, by painting his frames and creating intermediate zones where the painting never quite comes up against the world. One of the ways in which the painter encapsulated his small intimate and private worlds was through his very individual use of framing. He framed his pictures with old frames he scavenged or bought and then painted across them to both blur this boundary but also to protect his paintings from too much exposure to other things.

To enter into his work we need to be able to experience not only that it is indeed paint he is using but also that he is conveying something very real. The framing helps to focus us into the painting but because it is also part of the painting it eases us into a different way of looking.

> I sometimes go to immense lengths to, as it were, fortify them before they leave the studio. The more evanescent the emotion I want to convey, the thicker the panel, the heavier the framing, the more

elaborate the border so that this delicate thing will remain protected and intact.

(Auping, 1995: 20)

There is a sense of fragility and terror expressed here in case that which he has created will all too easily be destroyed or lost.

When I returned home from the Tate exhibition and next saw my patient who was feeling suicidal, something had moved on in the work. I knew that I was feeling less anxious about him and he seemed to have retreated back from an edge. It may be fanciful to think that understanding a bit more about how Hodgkin used his feeling sense as the base material for his art, all the while being aware of how delicate this process was, had in some way affected my therapeutic work in a positive way. I was certainly more aware of how any feeling state, however intense, may be temporary, a small moment in time, which will move past us and move on.

Chapter 14

The heretic

Art was creeping into and informing my psychotherapy practice and my work with patients. I became more aware of how my thoughts about psychoanalysis and art crossed over each other and sometimes aligned. I was beginning to appreciate that good art, like psychoanalysis, can be a heretical endeavour, going against the grain of the status quo and suggesting new ways of seeing the world and ourselves. Submitting oneself to psychotherapy or psychoanalysis has the intent of questioning both. It is not about a process of fitting in. All the artists that I have loved have been heretical to some extent, challenging norms and setting out their own unique view of the world. I could now see that the appeal of psychoanalysis and art was that they both wished to disrupt and question. It seemed that they might have similar aims in view.

There were some struggles in my consulting room that were becoming especially intriguing to me and which I felt I might understand more fully through art rather than through psychoanalytic theory. Many of my female patients who were performers, writers or artists had expressed difficulties in getting started in their work and brought all their frustrations about feeling blocked into the consulting room. They seemed to find that there were obstacles constantly in their way, whether from outside of themselves or of their own making. I began a project in which I considered whether men and women had similar or very different issues when struggling with their creativity. My female patients seemed to be telling me that their difficulties revolved around their need to remain acceptable as women. These ideas eventually turned into a book about how certain successful female artists were able to express the destructive as well as the creative side of their artistic expression and how by doing this they seemed to be able to break through these obstacles (Miller, 2008).

One of the artists I studied was Louise Bourgeois, who was in a way an obvious choice. She was a dynamic, visceral and rather formidable woman who straddled the 20th and 21st centuries with an enormous body of work. She was known for her fierce determination and her interest in sexuality, gender and female experience. I had first seen her work at the large retrospective at Tate Modern in 1999, and I was fascinated by her apparent lack of concern about what the art world or the public thought of what she produced. She appeared fiercely independent, the mistress of her own trajectory and completely unaffected by the demands of the art world. She freely admitted that all her work was autobiographical and that she used the memories of her childhood and her relationships with her parents to psychologically fire up her creativity. Many of my female patients expressed the view that Bourgeois' work was immensely empowering for them.

The biographical details of Bourgeois' life are well known as she constantly referred to them herself, but they need briefly relating here. She was the middle child of French parents who ran a workshop in Paris on the Boulevard Saint-Germain where they restored medieval tapestries. Louise grew up surrounded by silk, threads and needles and all the intricacies of sewing. The formative and, as she describes it, the most traumatic event of her childhood was when a young English governess, Sadie Richmond, was taken into the household to instruct the children and subsequently became her father's mistress, and then stayed in the house with the family for ten years. Sadie's presence in the house was accepted by Mme. Bourgeois but, as a consequence, Louise's mother suppressed her own anger about the relationship.

The artist referred frequently to this period of her childhood and revisited it in subsequent works about both her mother and father in which she explored her rage, the capacity of her mother for reparation and destruction, her sadistic fantasies against her father, her sexuality and her fascination with threads and sewing. As a young woman Bourgeois studied art at the Sorbonne and eventually married an art historian and moved to New York where she spent the rest of a very long life. She worked up until 2010 when she died at the age of 98.

For half her working life from the 1940s to the 1980s Bourgeois made her art in relative obscurity, but she kept on working. 'It was just that I had the feeling that the art scene belonged to the men and that I was in some way invading their domain. Therefore the work was done and hidden away' (Bourgeois, 1998: 112).

Once the artist started showing more of her work and became better known, she began to disseminate her own interpretations of how her childhood had affected her and how it was the source of much of her inspiration. She had a long psychoanalysis and she kept notes about her struggles with her jealousy, rage and her insomnia, notes which have come to light and been published since her death in 2010 (Bourgeois, 2012). Rather than allowing others to fish around in her history and explore the experiences and motivations behind her work she did this herself, frequently giving interviews where she offered Freudian interpretations of what her work meant and how it could be read. These interpretations were not always consistent but they provided a screen between her and the critics, behind which she could work in peace. The initial outward impression was that she was extremely open about her work and her motivations. It was as if she had already said all there was to be said about her creative sources and, by doing so, closed off other interpretations from art critics and journalists. If you are your own analyst and link your early traumas to your later creative work it is difficult for critics to have a say. It was as if Bourgeois removed others' ability to psychoanalyze her work – an extremely clever and protective move on her part.

I needed some illustrations of Bourgeois' work for the chapter I was writing and she agreed to let me have them on a CD. During a trip to New York I went to her studio in the old meatpacking district of Manhattan to collect it. The area was a rather bleak industrial area of large warehouse buildings that had been purloined by artists who needed big spaces. I was excited at the thought of seeing inside the studio and pressed the bell with anticipation. As the door opened an ethereal voice from the intercom told me to come up the stairs. At the top of the stairs I was met by the assistant who handed me the CD. All doors to the studio were firmly shut and it was obvious that this was going to be a one-way and two-word conversation, which consisted of a 'thank you' on my part and a replying nod. Afterwards I realized that my hope of seeing inside the studio or even seeing Bourgeois herself was completely unrealistic, but that it had been based on the idea that the artist was an open book and that therefore she would be happy to reveal herself to me. This was of course my fantasy, but one that she had encouraged in her own overt explorations of her artistic motivations.

Before writing my chapter I had visited the retrospective exhibition of Bourgeois' work at Tate Modern a couple of times, to try and take on board the wide variety of her output. Drawings, sculptures of varying sizes in bronze, wood and plaster, sewn objects, constructed rooms, vitrines and mirrors were all part of the eclectic body of her work. By then she had been producing work for over fifty years. The first work which I could not avoid and which filled part of the turbine hall was the gigantic bronze and steel spider titled *Maman*.

I was thrilled with the size of this work, which seemed to dominate the hall – not a small feat. It was exhilarating to think that a woman could have made such an enormous sculpture and taken up so much space. *Maman* was beautiful but also predatory. Spiders are the insects that can terrify and render phobic many people, most frequently women. A fear of spiders can be passed on from mother to daughter and the idea of standing under a giant spider would have been impossible for many women. Female spiders procreate and weave and kill.

I had, a few days before, been bitten by a large and very hairy spider that had found its way into the bedroom and the two red bites on my hand were still throbbing. Despite this I found this spider exhilarating. The black insect crouched in the turbine hall on her bent spindly legs. Her pregnant body hung down like a filled sack. Through the perforated bronze of her abdomen I could see a collection of white marble eggs glistening. Once I was standing underneath this body I felt protected, but I also had the strange sensation that she might collapse on me and devour me. Could I trust her? On balance I probably couldn't, as she was potentially both a devouring and protecting mother.

By calling the piece *Maman* Bourgeois was referring to her own mother, or to herself as a mother. The artist said she associated spiders with protection and repair, 'I came from a family of repairers ... If you bash into the web of a spider she doesn't get mad, she weaves and repairs it' (Blomberg, 2007), and she added that her own associations to spiders were the words 'deliberate, patient, soothing, reasonable, dainty, neat' (Morris, 2003: 66).

I had read these pronouncements from the artist about her own creative sources but in this case it seemed to me as if she was trying to hide the predatory nature of her sculpture. The experience of standing under *Maman* was exhilarating because of her size and power, and the potential threat of being eaten was part of this excitement. Prior to seeing a lot of her work, the creative fictions from the artist had woven their own spidery web around me and wrapped me in a cocoon of anticipation. I was delighted with her psychological understanding and her willingness to share it and what she had said about this sculpture obviously contained *a* truth. But by the time I was standing under *Maman* with its enormous weight pressing down on me, I began to wonder whether Bourgeois was only able to use her rage and aggression in her art by hiding these emotions behind a feminine screen of weaving and repair. For a female sculptor to make a work that dominated the turbine hall suggested to me that she *was* able to inhabit and use her aggression to further her creativity and maybe the danger for her was to acknowledge this.

The Jungian Sue Austin, in her book *Women's Aggressive Fantasies*, quotes a painter called Isla: 'When I paint I feel omnipotent. I think it's the closest I'll ever come to "God" or a higher being. Or maybe it's what men feel like ... I've created so I can move forward' (Austin, 2005: 123). Making art introduces women to a sense of their power. Instead of Bourgeois offering *Maman* as a containing space for others, which the women in my consulting room were so used to doing for their families and friends, the artist had become her own agent and was using the vast space as if there were no limits to how much room she could take up in the world. She seemed to be living comfortably with her aggression albeit suggesting otherwise.

This need to create as a woman, combined with the fear of how any creation would be received, were the conflicting emotions coming from my patients, but they also strongly reminded me of my teenage and early adult years when I felt that my rage against patriarchy and society's ideas of how women should be couldn't be expressed through my painting or writing without dire consequences. Now I was discovering that my female patients' fears about what would happen to them if they allowed their creativity full rein were being reflected in Bourgeois' words, which expressed her fragility. This did not hold her back in her art because she seemed to have found a way to deflect attacks when she was actually giving free rein to what might be seen as the un-feminine and more destructive parts of her nature. I began to see that I might be able to feed this into my work in the consulting room.

After the spider had exerted its powers over me, I moved on from the turbine hall to the upper galleries of the Tate where another important but much earlier work, made in 1968, was displayed. *Filette* is a larger-than-life-size latex and plaster sculpture of male genitals (Figure 14.1). It was hanging from a wire in the ceiling in the middle of the gallery so it was possible to walk all the way round it and to watch it move slightly in the displaced air.

My first response was to think of this as a rather violent castration, as there was no sense of the body to which this sexual part might have been attached. The male member was hanging like an offering to the gods, as if

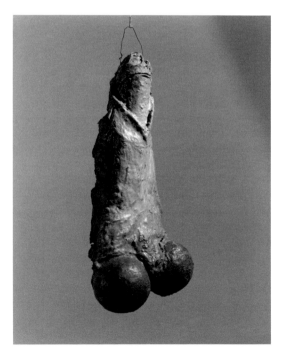

Figure 14.1 Louise Bourgeois, *Filette*, 1968, latex over plaster, hanging piece. Collection of Museum of Modern Art, New York.

© The Easton Foundation/DACS, London. Photo © Allan Finkelman.

female rage had just carried out a tabooed fantasy. Yet it also made me think of virility symbols. Like a carved yoni stone in India, it was there to bring fertility to both people and the land.

There was also a strange ambiguity about the sexuality expressed by this piece. Was it a virile male member or was it an expression of the masculine in the feminine as the sculpture was also suggestive of the roundness of the female form? From some angles it seemed to reference both male and female body parts. There was a contrasexuality inherent in the work and in the name the artist had given it, *Filette (Little Girl)*. Was this to diffuse the inherent aggression of the work or was she suggesting that the feminine could be present here too and that women could also inhabit and own some of this male power? After the exhibition I came across the photograph that Robert Mapplethorpe took of the artist wearing her monkey-skin jacket and holding *Filette* tenderly under her arm. She is looking towards the camera with a conspiratorial smile.

'When I carry a phallus like that in my arms, well, it seems like a nice little object, it's certainly not an object I would wish to harm, that's clear. The niceness is directed towards men' (Bernadec, 1996: 67). Yet again, as with her other pronouncements, Bourgeois is acknowledging ambiguity here, as it is clear that she is the one in control. I loved this photograph. It epitomized for me the issues around power and sexuality that women faced, and how in order to be creative women had to embrace their own phallic power. Bourgeois does this with *Filette*, but tempers any aggressive response there might be to that by insisting that the sculpture is a reminder of the vulnerability of both men and women. 'I remember a model in life-drawing class at the Beaux-Arts getting an erection. He was embarrassed and I was amazed at how vulnerable he really was' (Bernadec, 1996: 81).

A year after she made *Filette*, Bourgeois continued her fascination with body parts by making *Femme-Couteau (Knife Woman)* (Figure 14.2). This small sculpture is carved out of a piece of pink marble. The female body is knife-like and headless.

It is without doubt a representation of the feminine, but it is sharp as well as rounded and, I imagined, could be used as a weapon to pierce a body, although the forms also suggested flowers and leaves from the natural world. 'In the *Femme-Couteau*, the woman turns into a blade, she is defensive. She identifies with the penis to defend herself ... We are all vulnerable in some way, and we are all male-female' (Bernadec, 1996: 86).

A couple of years after seeing the retrospective of her work at the Tate I came across a small exhibition of her more recent pieces in Edinburgh. *Stiches in Time* featured some of her sewn and stuffed objects, feminine in their realization but many full of pain and anguish and all made when the artist was in her nineties. There were various stuffed and sewn heads, some encased in glass boxes, some freestanding, and these heads were full of terror and sensitive intricacy. *Untitled* was a small head made from aluminium and

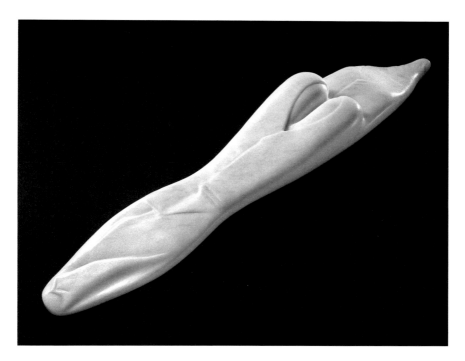

Figure 14.2 Louise Bourgeois, *Femme Couteau*, 1969–1970, pink marble.
© The Easton Foundation/DACS, London. Photo © Allan Finkelman.

tapestry (Figure 14.3). Blue eyes stared out of a decorated face and the mouth was open to show a red gash. The tapestry had been carefully moulded round the form to follow the woven pattern. There was also a roughness about how the material was sewn together, almost as if the face has suffered surgery of some kind or been bandaged to protect its wounds.

This head reminded me of a Greek mask, a mask showing anguish and pain frozen in time. As I looked closer I could see that the pieces of cloth were put together with tiny stiches, like those used by Bourgeois' mother in the repairing of the tapestries. Stiches carried for the artist a possibility of reparation of the past and making new again. Here was an original object now remade into another form, and through this re-making a reparation of part of her childhood had taken place. The artist was returning again to the themes of her early life, reforming a tapestry into a head, a head that then seemed full of its own memories.

In one sense this was simply a piece of tapestry stretched over an aluminium form, but it suggested a head without a body speaking from the

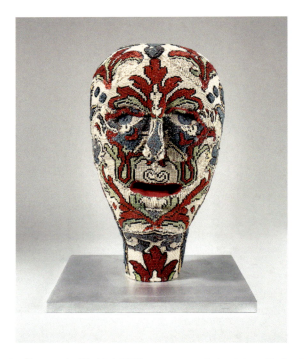

Figure 14.3 Louise Bourgeois, *Untitled*, 2002, tapestry and aluminium. Collection Glenstone Foundation.
© The Easton Foundation/DACS, London. Photo © Christopher Burk.

grave. It captured for me the pain and anguish of some of my patients and the difficulties women artists have to overcome to be able to express their most powerful feelings. Again Bourgeois was expressing her rage and confusion, but this time through the use of soft materials. A male artist might have made this form out of stone or bronze. Bourgeois was using materials that were close to her heart and which could be sewn and stretched rather than chipped at. This sculpture was a powerful, feminine work with a soft exterior but with a hard metal structure inside. It reminded me of the Bolivian aguayos I had seen so many years before and my sense that they were a protection and armour for the women who made and wore them. The women of the Altiplano were not displaying female rage in the same way that Bourgeois was but they were using their art as a symbol of their power and independence from men.

I was disturbed and moved by this head. I wanted to live with it and wondered in reality whether, if given the chance, I would have been able to bear it. Bourgeois' work conveys a world of female choice, power and aggression. It explores a struggle for the feminine in all its murderous and sadistic elements as well as its loving ones. Her words, though, speak of a vulnerability driven by childhood trauma and these words and interpretations do not allow the status quo to be disrupted in the way that her work suggests. She seemed to have found a way to protect herself against the male art establishment by suggesting that her work was entirely to do with her family relationships and therefore not the threat that it might otherwise have been seen as. In reality her work is about how powerful and creative women can be if released from cultural constraints.

By the time Bourgeois was in her eighties and nineties and up until her death her fame protected her from outright attacks and she became more outspoken and confident. Although physically frail, she held gatherings at her New York home for other artists to talk about their work and receive her opinions. The British sculptor Richard Long, who attended some of these afternoon sessions, described them as 'seances'; she had become the *Master* (Long, 2010). For a contemporary artist, let alone a female one, to exert this kind of influence in her lifetime was revolutionary. This influence was a direct result of Bourgeois' formidable and startling creativity, but it also related to her ability throughout her lifetime to keep a tight control over both the interpretation of her work and her own biographical text.

To those patients of mine who were admirers of Bourgeois, I reflected to them that her ability to weave a web around herself had given her the essential protection she needed to be able to then express her aggression and destruction as well as her love. She didn't have to hold herself back because of fears about how her work would be received. She presented a wonderful example of hiding in plain sight.

As well as encouraging and spurring my own patients on, Bourgeois was also enormously influential in my own creative endeavours. I had admired other women artists in the past and now I was beginning to discover contemporary women artists who excited me. Bourgeois seemed to grasp the heretical nature of art with such aplomb, at the same time as acknowledging that this was a dangerous position to take. She spurred me on.

Chapter 15

Walking

After many years working as a Jungian analyst I began to develop pains in my neck and back. It seemed obvious to me that these were brought on by sitting down all day in the same chair and in the same position whilst listening to my patients. Whilst they moved between chair and couch, got up to go to the loo, fidgeted, stretched, yawned, cried, sat on the floor, crept under blankets and showed me in a multitude of physical ways how they were feeling, I continued to sit still, occasionally turning slightly towards the couch or crossing or uncrossing my legs. In breaks between sessions I tried to go for short walks and I started a regular Pilates class, but my body complained constantly and I felt more and more constrained by my sedentary life. My dreams at the time seemed to be full of people walking. They were on long walks, hard walks and constantly in movement. Occasionally I seemed to be allowed to join them in the dreams, but difficulties were put in my way. Despite trying to enact my dreams by taking myself for walks when I could, the nightly perambulations continued – a sure sign that I had not registered something in my unconscious. After a while I stopped taking the dreams so concretely and thought more about what the dream-walking was representing.

I had been seeing patients for almost twenty years and become used to carrying their stories and their emotions around with me; for that is what therapists do, they embody both the conscious and unconscious in the psyche of others. Part of the therapeutic training is to enable us to do this and to look after ourselves at the same time, yet once you are in the world of the unconscious nothing is that clear cut. Feelings, images and reactions were not under my conscious control; however many boundaries I put around my work, there were leaks into both my conscious and unconscious life. Patients' emotions sometimes infected me deeply and then it felt very difficult to remain apart. I found that I carried around their sadness or joy and after a while their personalities and characters seemed to be an ongoing part of myself. However much I filled my time away from my work with writing, seeing friends or looking at art, those lives and emotions were always still with me.

Often I picked up emotions that had not been voiced by the patient and I struggled to disentangle and name them. Sometimes I was aware of worrying about a patient because of their precarious state of health. Other times they were simply in my thoughts because I was fond of them. Either way all my patients found a space to reside inside me. If the therapeutic work is going to be helpful this kind of containment by the therapist is essential. I didn't begrudge it, as one of the attractions of being a psychotherapist was how exposed I was to the fascinating internal lives of others. But I did begin to wonder whether the walking dreams were a metaphor for being freer in my mind as well as my body.

I slowly allowed myself the surprising thought of no longer seeing patients. I began to wonder what it would be like to have none to think about and how much that might free up space to consider where I wanted to go next. This was a radical idea for me as I had imagined that I would continue working until old age. The reality however seemed to be somewhat different. Although I still needed to earn, I began to feel myself straining to be free and to reclaim my internal world for my own introspection and possible creativity. After much thought and trying out the idea on colleagues, I gave my patients two years' notice and began reducing my practice. Those two years were difficult, as I frequently regretted the decision and wondered how I could bear to stop the work with some of the patients I felt most attached to, but I persisted.

Soon after saying goodbye to my last patients, I made a visit to Tate Britain and was stunned by a work by the British land artist Richard Long (Figure 15.1). The floor of the long central hall of Tate Britain was covered by a perambulating china clay path, which Long had poured from a watering can. The white flowing line travelled from one of the arches and along the black tiled floor, like a twisting colon, obeying invisible lines down either side but otherwise filling the hall like a river seen from space. It was an energetic life form with a certainty and delight in its own process. I wanted to trace my steps along this exhilarating maze as if the walking of it might bring about some kind of revelation. The work seemed exuberant and wild and showed through the spills and reverses that Long had allowed the liquid clay to find its own form and obey its own rules.

It was as if the artist had encouraged the clay to do its own thing. *White Water Line* embodied art, the natural environment and walking in one curvaceous swirl, and I delighted in this freedom of expression. Walking up and down the length of it I felt liberated. Long had obviously not felt constrained by marking the illustrious art gallery in this way.

I was intrigued enough to go, two years later, to a retrospective of Long's work again at the Tate. Maybe I went with a friend, maybe not. The details of the day have disappeared, leaving behind an intense visual and sensory experience. The exhibition covered a lifetime of Long's work, photographs, wall paintings, floor sculptures, text works and map works all related to the central preoccupation of his life – walking.

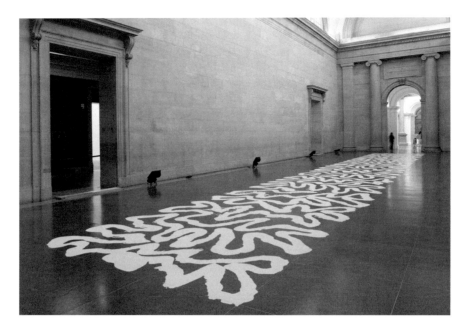

Figure 15.1 Richard Long, *White Water Line*, 2007.
Courtesy of the artist and Tate. Photo © Tate.

Richard Long's work defies categories, as he has throughout his career invented his own art forms. Whilst still a student he made a line through a field of daisies by walking up and down it. He then took a photograph and *A Line Made by Walking* catapulted him into the forefront of contemporary art at the age of twenty-two. He is referred to as a land artist, a conceptual artist and a sculptor. His work is frequently based in the landscape, but he also makes work from natural elements specifically for galleries. A lot of his work made in the landscape is only seen through the photographs he takes, as these works are often in isolated places and then the works disappear back into the landscape from which they have come. Nature reclaims the grass, earth or stones Long has temporarily co-opted. Much of the artist's gallery work on floors and walls and made with china clay or mud is cleaned off after the exhibition is over. The art that remains are the photographs and his sculptural pieces made of rocks, stones and pebbles.

Long is an instinctual artist and waits for the right moment and right place to make a work. He sets off on long walks for days and weeks and then waits until a place resonates with him. He then moves rocks or places stones or piles up sticks and takes a photograph of what he has made before moving on. The land and the landscape are his studio. 'That's the reason I'm not a studio artist, because being in the real world, being always in landscape is a much better way for all these things to happen; so I put myself at a fantastic advantage in a way' (Long, 2010).

Going on extensive walks not only exposes him to a variety of landscapes but also enables Long to enter into a specific state of mind. As Wordsworth knew, walking can induce a creative space in the mind. The writer Rebecca Solnit says in her book on the history of walking that the speed of walking is the speed of 'the mind at three miles an hour' (Solnit, 2002: 14). The rhythm of the body walking is the same as the natural rhythm of the mind in a state of free-floating attention. Whilst walking there is a reduction in conscious attention, a letting go of concerns and idle thoughts, and the mind is able to slip into a different gear, to enter a liminal space where images and ideas are more accessible. This slipping of gears was something I was aware of happening sometimes in my consulting room, but when there I was in this space for the sole purpose of thinking and reacting more deeply to another person. Long was showing me that physical movement could also bring about this state, which could then be harnessed for one's own creative thinking. Walking is indicative of a certain freedom, a freedom to go where one wishes. My walking dreams had been suggesting to me that I needed to be less confined physically but also mentally; that I needed to be able to walk around in my head.

The photographs of the work Long makes on his solitary walks are the only signs we have of this intense walking and making activity. There was a photograph of one of these works in the Tate exhibition that I became transfixed by. *Circle in Africa. Mulanje Mountain Malawi* was a black and white photo of charred cacti that had been burnt in lightning storms and which the artist had rearranged in a circle. The landscape looked like it had been devastated by a forest fire. The lowering clouds moving fast above the land presaged rain. From out of this devastation the artist had created a circle of burnt cacti suggesting a ritual wholeness or healing of some kind. As I stood in the sterile white-walled Tate I could smell the rich mixture of earth and the burning of vegetation that I had previously only encountered in my trips to the African bush.

I kept breathing in and out expecting this strange sensation to disappear but there it still was. My sense of smell was picking up something conveyed by a visual image. I felt I was there in that landscape and experiencing the work with all my senses. The photograph seemed to be able to transmit more than the recording of a temporary sculpture made from charred cacti. Everything had come together, the brooding clouds, the charred trees, the man-made circle – nature and the artist had met in a 'decisive moment' – the phrase the photographer Henri Cartier Bresson used to describe the coming together of an idea and its visual form (Cartier Bresson, 1952).

Other works in the retrospective show fascinated me too, the exuberant circles of slate and stone, the enigmatic text works about walks the artist had made, and the sheer exhilaration of *White Water Falls* (Figure 15.2), which dripped down a black painted wall like a mist of water coming over a waterfall. Visitors were walking up and down beside this wall as if experiencing some natural phenomenon – a thick mist of air-borne water above and a falling sheet of water below. It looked as if the watery flows were disappearing into the air-conditioning vents in the gallery floor.

I found it painful to think that this beautiful wall painting would be whitewashed out at the end of the exhibition. When I later interviewed Long I asked him about this constant loss of his work, either by man-made whitewash or natural elimination, and he seemed resigned to its ephemeral nature. As I had just found it hard myself going through the process of giving up a part of my professional life, I experienced this ease with the natural dissolution and destruction of all things, even if they had been created by oneself, as very refreshing. It suggested to me that Long valued the creative moment and the timing of his art more than the end product. It also helped me to trust in the work I had done with my patients as an entity that had been valuable and had passed, and that I could start to believe that the space I had now given myself for new explorations was valuable.

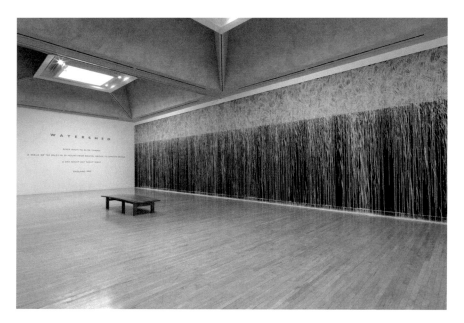

Figure 15.2 Richard Long, *White Water Falls*, 2009, Exhibition: Heaven and Earth, Tate. Courtesy of the artist. Photo © Tate.

There seemed to be many things in Long's work that were reflecting my need to find a space for my own creative ideas. I now had extensive periods of time to use as I wished, so I started making trips to track down Long's works, or at least those that were accessible and permanent features in the landscape. I discovered that Roche Court near Salisbury had a sculpture made of flint on permanent display in their Sculpture Park. Roche Court lies in the verdant rolling Wiltshire countryside, a far cry from Malawi, but I was interested to see whether the work responded to and reflected the landscape in the same kind of way as the photograph in the Tate had. Beside a beautiful Georgian house *Tame Buzzard Line* lay below a flowering lavender hedge (Figure 15.3).

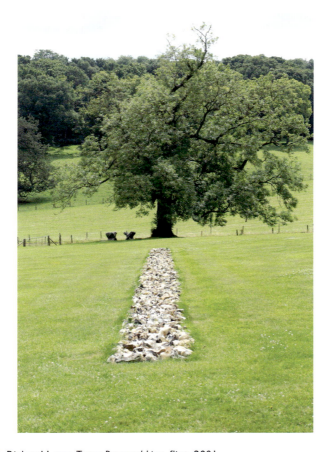

Figure 15.3 Richard Long, *Tame Buzzard Line*, flint, 2001.
Courtesy the artist and New Art Centre Roche Court Sculpture Park. Photo © the author.

The grass of the sloping field was cut short, and rising a few inches above the surface of the grass was a long line of flint-stones about two feet wide. Once I had descended a few feet to the level of the field I could see that the line pointed directly towards a large ash tree. When I walked to the other end, turned around and allowed my eyes to follow the upward curve of the smooth green sward, I saw that the line pointed to another large ash tree just below the level of the house. The sculpture highlighted the fall of the field and seemed to describe in its straight falling swoop the movement of a bird above it. A buzzard flying back from one tree to another would have etched the same line across the field with its shadow. It was as if the artist had intuited this movement of the bird when first staring at the open field, and simply made it more conscious by laying down his flints so that we could see what was already there, something previously hidden in an unconscious layer of the landscape, in the *underland*.

This long line of flints was strangely satisfying. I felt like saying, 'Of course, yes', as if a part of the landscape had been opened up and revealed. It seemed that Long was both responding to the contours and lines of the landscape and then had peeled away a façade and for a moment I could see things as they really were. This was not just a mown field with a beautiful ash tree but a marker registering through the flints the buzzard's repeated swooping flight.

My tracking of Long's work then took me to Norfolk where in the grounds of Houghton Hall there was a large slate sculpture acquired by the Marquess of Cholmondeley for the grand vista in front of his imposing house. The day was damp and there was a heavy grey Norfolk sky hanging over the vast mown acreage. From a distance *Full Moon Circle* looked like a circular pond cut into the grass, its surface glistening in the rain (Figure 15.4). As I got closer I could see that the shimmering surface was broken up by waves of dark grey slate tucked under each other like the scales on the back of an armadillo. I then found that I was walking round it clockwise, leading with my right shoulder as I circled the waves of slate. This curving movement brought back a body memory from a couple of years previously. The last time I had edged round a large circular object had been in India.

To show due reverence, Buddhist stupas should be walked round in a clockwise direction, so that the right side of the body, the unpolluted side, is closest to the building. This memory appeared apt as the circle had induced in me a meditative state. As I circled the sculpture a couple more times the rain began to fall more insistently and the expansive Norfolk sky became black and thunderous. As the sky grew darker the wet slate turned violet and the surrounding green lawn became iridescent.

On that day, in that weather, there was an otherness to my experience of the work. It was not a religious experience but it was spiritual in that it connected me deeply into the place I was standing in. I was intensely aware of being alive in the moment beside this dark circle and in front of the slightly forbidding edifice of Houghton Hall. *Full Moon Circle* had the effect of gathering

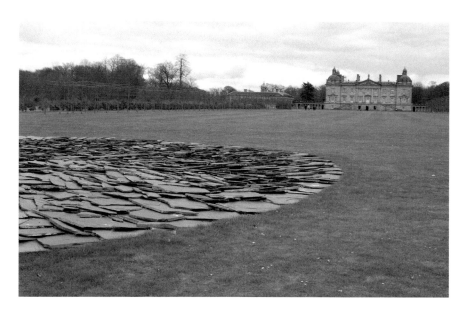

Figure 15.4 Richard Long, *Full Moon Circle*, slate, 2004.
Courtesy the artist and Houghton Hall, Norfolk. Photo © the author.

me up and connecting me into that open green ground in Norfolk in a way in which the landscape by itself had not done. I had seen through the work to something beyond it and in so doing I had felt a deep connection with the landscape.

Long is an artist who presents a world where all is not as it appears and suggests that if we absorb and look closely we may register other ways of seeing that we may not have been aware of before. He is not a sculptor in the original sense of the word. He doesn't chip away at slabs of marble or cast objects in bronze. He gets his materials to speak without carving or breaking them in any way. He is not aggressive with his stones or slate, but is sensitive to their properties. By rearranging them in circles, lines and spirals he seems to discover a different mode of expression and a multitude of associations. The artist Michael Craig-Martin said of him: 'It's always struck me as very interesting about how much Richard is able to get from a material while being extremely passive with it. He never forces it to do anything, he kind of unblocks something in the material' (Craig-Martin, 1990).

Circling *Full Moon Circle* I was reminded of the sharpness and darkness of the wet slate roofs of the outbuildings on my uncle's Welsh farm, where it seemed to rain whenever I was there. Sometimes on special nights I'd be called out to stand in my pyjamas and wellingtons under a dripping slate roof to watch a cow being born. Slate was an intrinsic part of the buildings and the land on the farm. Walking round *Full Moon Circle* also took me back to India and the significance there, in that hot land, of the circle as both a religious and a containing symbol. All these associations, Welsh slate, Norfolk sky, Buddhist stupas combined for me into a new experience of Norfolk, the vast flatness of the land and the lowering sky had been mirrored and picked up by the circular sculpture and made into something intensely personal.

The more I found of the artist's work, the more I became obsessed with my search. I was keen to experience, as often as possible, that sense of losing myself in front of Long's art. The process of tracking down his work became my *walking* experience, as I felt opened out by contact with mud, clay, stones and slate. Long seemed unconstrained in his use of the natural world, which he treated with reverence and love, at the same time as constantly asking it to reveal something more, as if *out there* there was an infinite source of creative possibilities. I had been absorbed and fascinated with my therapy work, but it had narrowed my gaze as I had immersed myself in the imaginative exploration of the minds of others. I hoped that I had been able to unblock creative possibilities for some of my patients but now I needed my gaze to look outwards again – to experience art as a direct relationship between me and the paint or marble or stone and to be unaffected by my absorption in the minds of others.

Chapter 16

Afterword

Sixty years ago, the psychoanalyst Marion Milner, through the exploration of her own artistic process, came to the conclusion that,

> a work of art, whatever its content, or subject, whether a recognizable scene or object or abstract pattern, must be an externalization, through its shapes and lines and colours, of the unique psycho-physical rhythm of the person making it. Otherwise it will have no life in it whatever, for there is no other source for its life.
>
> (Milner, 1957: 163)

Milner understood that this rhythm, as she called it, was essential for a work of art to live and have a presence in the world. She also understood that this rhythm was vulnerable to attack.

Psychoanalysts and psychotherapists have a long history of co-opting artists and their work as subjects for psychological examination. Freud began this with his paper on Leonardo da Vinci in 1910 (Freud, 1990), and then in 1934 Jung wrote about Picasso (Jung, 1966: 135–141). More recently Louise Bourgeois has provided psychoanalysts with clinical material that can be picked apart (Kuspit, 2012; Williams, 2012). These essays have often had the intention of exploring the relationship between disturbance and creativity. The writers have been inclined to think about the work of artists as an attempt to defend themselves against a discrepancy between their inner and outer worlds and that, as a result, art is a process of reparation for the artist. This may well be true in some instances but, as Maclagan suggests, such psychological interpretations of art can be destructive as they 'can split the aesthetic level of a painting from its "deep" unconscious meaning, divorcing the aesthetic and the psychological' (Maclagan, 2001: 13). Once this has happened art loses its essential magic, its ability to move, seduce and excite us; it has simply been turned into an object of therapeutic exploration and separated off from its own internal life, the blood of the work no longer flows.

Afterword

As a psychotherapist my interest in art and artists has been to try and respond directly to the life of the work. I have tried not to dissect the work, and separate the psychology of the artist from the art they create, nor to see the work as a result of the artist's pathology, and I may have only been partly successful in this. However I hope in this book that I have managed to convey my experience of art through my own emotional and physical responses, to have observed and described my own internal world as it responds to the aesthetic expression of the internal world of another. Artists enable us, as those who look, to better understand ourselves. They hold an enormous creative potential for us all to tap into and, if we so wish, to use as a form of self-analysis. Like a reflecting mirror they show us more of ourselves, what we are, what we are not and to what we might aspire.

Good artists generously present their work to us for use as a method of self-exploration in any way we may wish. To do this they risk inhabiting a space of dissolved boundaries, where certainties are no longer certain, and this is where they live and breathe and work. It can be a world of disturbance, distress and violent emotions but this is a reflection of all our internal worlds, not simply those of creative artists. They expose themselves to the rigors and dangers of this liminal place to show us how we and the world may not be quite as we think they are and in so doing they take enormous risks. From my contacts and interviews with artists and those patients who are artists that I have had the privilege to work with, I have seen how their drive to create is intrinsic to their personalities and their psyches. It is often as if they have no choice but to make and explore and to go on making and exploring. Their creativity enables us to follow them in their search and to discover ourselves along the way.

This book reflects a small part of my own explorations in art and how these have linked up to my development, my emotions and my growing sense of self. When I had seen the world through eyes transformed by Renoir blue paint or I had marvelled at the intensity of *Red Studio* these childhood responses remained so vivid because they had helped me to explore who I might become. They taught me to look and to feel and to consider my feelings. In midlife I had sought out art, sometimes as a reassurance and sometimes for the relief it gave me, and always for creative encouragement. More recently I have used art to better understand the unconscious aspects of myself and my patients. Great art still has the power to make my inner world vibrate.

*

This is not the end I hope. At any time now a scene may repeat itself. I'll walk into a gallery and search out a painting I want to see, or I might notice one for the first time and wonder why I have not looked at it before. I might travel far to see a canvas that I have only seen in reproduction, and thrill as I did as a child to encounter the *real thing*. In all these scenes I will stand and look, and maybe become more aware of how the painter felt as they worked and how I am now feeling as I take the work in. If I am lucky a sense of time will evaporate, and I'll enter that zone of enchantment, where paint and my body become one, boundaries dissolve and I find I have crossed into a new territory where I can experience myself in relation to another's psyche and as a result can grow and develop.

Bibliography

Alcantara, I. 2011. *Frida Kahlo and Diego Rivera*. London: Prestel Publishing.
Ankori, G. 2002. *Imaging Her Selves: Frida Kahlo's Poetics of Identity and Fragmentation*. Connecticut: Praeger.
Auping, M. 1995. *Howard Hodgkin Paintings*. London: Thames and Hudson.
Austin, S. 2005. *Women's Aggressive Fantasies: A Post-Jungian Exploration of Self-Hatred, Love and Agency*. London: Routledge.
Bailey, M. 2003. *Vermeer*. London: Phaidon Press.
Bernadec, M.-L. 1996. *Louise Bourgeois*. Paris: Flammarion.
Blomberg, C. 2007. 'Interview with Louise Bourgeois', in *Louise Bourgeois*, ed. Francis Morris. London, p. 272.
Bourgeois, L. 1998. *Louise Bourgeois: Destruction of the Father/Reconstruction of the Father: Writings and Interviews 1923–1997*. M-l. Bernadec & H-U. Obrist (Eds). London: Violette Editions.
Bourgeois, L. 2012. *The Return of the Repressed. Vol 2. Psychoanalytic Writings*. London: Violette.
Boyd White, J. 2001. *The Edge of Meaning*. Chicago, IL: University of Chicago Press.
Brennan, T. 2004. *The Transmission of Affect*. Ithaca, NY: Cornell University Press.
Cartier Bresson, H. 1952. *The Decisive Moment*. Göttingen: Steidl Verlag.
Craig-Martin, M. 1990. *Third Opinion*, BBC Radio Three. 6.11.1990.
D'Alessandro, S. and Edenfield, J. 2010. *Matisse: Radical Invention 1913–1917*. New Haven, CT: Yale University Press.
Danchev, A. 2012. *Cezanne: A Life*. London: Profile Books Ltd.
Della Francesca, P.P. 1474–1482. *On Perspective in Painting*. Manuscript in Biblioteca Palatina in Parma.
Ede, H.S. 1971. *Savage Messiah*. London: Gordon Fraser.
Elkins, J. 1996. *The Object Stares Back: On the Nature of Seeing*. London: A Harvest Book.
Elkins, J. 1999. *What Painting Is*. Abingdon: Routledge.
Flam, J.D. 1973. *Matisse on Art*. London: Phaidon.
Freeman, D. 2012. *Art's Emotions: Ethics, Expression and Aesthetic Experience*. Durham: Acumen Publishing.
Freud, S. 1990. *Leonardo da Vinci and a Memory of His Childhood*. London: W.W. Norton and Co.
Gayford, M. 2007. *The Yellow House: Van Gogh, Gauguin and Nine Turbulent Weeks in Arles*. London: Penguin.

Gilot, F. 1990. *Matisse and Picasso*. London: Bloomsbury.
Graham-Dixon, A. 1994. *Howard Hodgkin*. London: Thames and Hudson.
Gregory, G. 2015. *The Studio: A Psychoanalytic Legacy*. London: Free Association Publishing.
Harrison, C. 2005. *Painting the Difference: Sex and Spectator in Modern Art*. Chicago: University of Chicago Press.
Hepworth, B. 1966. *Drawings from a Sculptor's Landscape*. London: Cory, Adams and Mackay.
Hodgkin, H. 1991. *About My Collection*. www.HowardHodgkin.com
Hood, W. 1993. *Fra Angelico at San Marco*. New Haven, CT: Yale University Press.
Hustvedt, S. 2005. *Mysteries of the Rectangle: Essays on Painting*. New York: Princeton Architectural Press.
Jung, C.G. 1966. *The Spirit in Man, Art and Literature*. Princeton, NJ: Princeton University Press.
Jung, C.G. 1970. *Psychology and Religion*. Princeton, NJ: Princeton University Press.
Jung, C.G. 1971. *Psychological Types. CW6*. London: Routledge.
Jung, C.G. 1984. *Dream Analysis*. The Seminars. London: Routledge and Kegan Paul.
Kalsched, D. 1996. *The Inner World of Trauma: Archetypal Defences of the Personal Spirit*. London: Routledge.
Kuspit, D. 2012. 'Symbolising Loss and Conflict: Psychoanalytic Process in Louise Bourgeois' Art', in *The Return of the Repressed*, Vol. 1, pp. 129–150. Ed. P. Larratt-Smith. London: Violette Editions.
Le Pichon, Y. 1985. *Le Monde du Douanier Rousseau*. Paris: Robert Laffont.
Long, R. 2010. Richard Long Interview with Juliet Miller [unpublished].
Maclagan, D. 2001. *Psychological Aesthetics: Painting, Feeling and Making Sense*. London: Jessica Kingsley.
Matisse, H. 1908. 'Notes of a Painter', in *La Grande Revue*. Paris: Bureau de la Grande Revue.
Miller, J. 2000. 'Training: Fears of Destruction and Creativity: Reflections on the Process of Becoming an Analyst', in *Harvest Journal for Jungian Studies*, Vol. 46, No. 2, pp. 53–69.
Miller, J. 2008. *The Creative Feminine and her Discontents: Psychotherapy, Art and Destruction*. London: Karnac.
Milner, M. 1957. *On Not Being Able to Paint*. New York: Penguin Putnam.
Morris, F. 2003. *Louise Bourgeois: Stiches in Time*. London: August. IMMA.
Morris, F. and Green, C. eds. 2006. *Henri Rousseau: Jungles in Paris*. London: Tate Publishing.
O'Keeffe, P. 2004. *Gaudier-Brzeska: An Absolute Case of Genius*. London: Allen Lane.
Parker, D. 2008. 'On Painting, Substance and Psyche', in *Psyche and the Arts: Jungian Approaches to Music, Architecture, Literature, Painting and Film*, pp. 45–55. Ed. S. Rowland. London: Routledge.
Paul, C. 2019. *Self Portrait*. London: Jonathan Cape.
Renoir, J. 1962. *Renoir My Father*. London: Collins.
Rose, J. 2002. *Demons and Angels: A Life of Jacob Epstein*. New York: Carroll and Graf.
Rousseau, P. 2006. 'The Magic of Images: Hallucination and Magnetic Reverie in the Work of Henri Rousseau', in *Henry Rousseau: Jungles in Paris*, pp. 191–203. Eds C. Green and F. Morris. London: Tate Publishing.

Serota, N. 2006. ed. *Howard Hodgkin: Interview with David Sylvester*. London: Tate Publishing.
Sidoli, M. 2000. *When the Body Speaks: The Archetypes in the Body*. London: Routledge.
Silber, E. 1996. *Gaudier-Brzeska: Life and Art*. London: Thames and Hudson.
Solnit, R. 2002. *Wanderlust: A History of Walking*. London: Verso.
Solnit, R. 2013. *The Faraway Nearby*. London: Granta.
Spurling, H. 1998. *The Unknown Matisse: A Life of Henri Matisse*. Vol. 1, 1869–1908. London: Hamish Hamilton.
Spurling, H. 2005. *Matisse the Master: A Life of Henri Matisse. The Conquest of Colour. 1909–1954*. London: Hamish Hamilton.
Townsend, P. 2019. *Creative States of Mind: Psychoanalysis and the Artist's Process*. Abingdon: Routledge.
Tucker, M. 1992. *Dreaming with Open Eyes: The Shamanic Spirit in Twentieth Century Art and Culture*. San Francisco: Aquarian/Harper.
Vollard, A. 1925. *Renoir: An Intimate Record*. New York: Alfred Knopf.
Vollard, A. 1936. *Recollections of a Picture Dealer*. London: Constable.
White, B.E. 1984. *Renoir: His Life Art and Letters*. New York: Harry Abrahams Inc.
Williams, M.H. 2012. 'The Child, the Container, and the Claustrum: The Artistic Vocation of Louise Bourgeois', in *The Return of the Repressed*, Vol. 1, pp. 31–44. ed. Philip Larratt-Smith. London: Violette Editions.
Wolf, B.J. 2001. *Vermeer and the Invention of Seeing*. Chicago: University of Chicago Press.

Index

Academie des Beaux-Arts 82
aesthetic: emotional 29; through form 45
aggression 41, 45, 110, 112
aguayo 51–54, 114
alchemy 87, 101
analysis 55, 83; self 4, 126
analytic training 64
Apollinaire, Guillaume 82
archetypes 82, 85
Arezzo 36
art: African 60; dissonance in 24; heretical 107, 115; Indian 104; indigenous 53; as language of loss 98; Pacific 60; silence in 91; stillness in 94
Austin, S. 110
Aymara 51, 52

Bagnold, Enid 4
beholder 100; *see also* gaze
birth: as coming into being 63; *see also* Epstein
body 58, 69; brain/body separation 43; response in 42, 81
borders 105
boundaries 76, 77, 86; as markers 77
Bourgeois, Louise 107–115, 125; *Femme Couteau* 112, 113; *Filette* 111, 112; *Maman* 109, 110; *Untitled* 112–114
Braque, Georges: *Still Life with Mandolin* 83
Bruegel, Pieter: *Landscape with the Fall of Icarus* 9–10
brush 13
brushstrokes 8, 16
Brzeska, Sophie 43

Cartier Bresson, Henri 119
Chardin, Jean 24

colour: as emotional state 24, 27, 28, 97, 99
conception 75
Corot, Jean 13
Cosimo de Medici 72
Courbet, Gustav 18
Craig-Martin, Michael 123
creativity 110; as battleground 29; as energy 27; as power 46

da Vinci, Leonardo 125
Degas, Edgar 2; *Helen Rouart in her Father's Study* 2–4
della Francesca, Piero 31–38; *The Baptism of Christ* 32; *The Legend of the True Cross* 36, 37; *Madonna del Parto* 34–36, 38; *The Nativity* 32–34, 37; *St Michael The Archangel* 32; *The Reception of the Queen of Sheba by King Solomon* 36
destruction 108, 120; as power 46
dreaming 83, 84
dreams 10, 55–56, 58, 79, 83, 85, 86
Dresden 88

Ede, Jim 39, 43; *Savage Messiah* 43
Elkins, J. 13, 28, 95, 101
empathy 42
enantiodromia 45
Epstein, Jacob 44, 55–63; *Birth* 62, 63; and 'primitive art' 60, 62; *Jacob and the Angel* 57, 58; *Mating Doves* 62; *St Michael and the Devil* 56

fantasies 79; sadistic 108
Les Fauves 29
First World War 43, 45
Flight, Claude 6

Fra Angelico 72–78; *The Annunciation* 73, 74, 76, 77
frames 11, 75, 105
framing 105
frescoes 72, 73, 75
Freud, S. 125

Gainsborough, Thomas: *Mr and Mrs Andrews* 7–8
Gaudier-Brzeska, Henri 40–46; *Bird Swallowing a Fish* 40–43, 46; *The Wrestlers* 45, 46
Gauguin, Paul 8
gaze 15, 16, 19, 79; male 19
Gilot, Françoise 29, 87
Goldsmidt, E. 26
Graham–Dixon, A. 104
grief 2

haptic 42; *see also* touch
Harrison, C. 19
Hirst, Damien: *The Physical Impossibility of Death in the Mind of Someone Living* 20
Hodgkin, Howard 28, 96–106; *Bombay Sunset* 101–103; *Clean Sheets* 98, 99, 101; *Dinner at Smith Square* 96, 97, 99
Hudson, William 62
Hustvedt, S. 95

The Impressionists 17, 18, 82
infertility 35, 62
International Congress of Physiological Psychology 85

Jung, C. G. 45, 83, 85; and alchemy 101; and Picasso 125; *Psychological Types* 45
Jungian analyst 4, 55, 63, 71

Kahlo, Frida 66–70; *Self Portrait with Braid* 69; *The Two Fridas* 66, 67
Kettle's Yard 39, 44, 45
Kipling, Rudyard 83

landscape: identity with 50; unconscious layer of 122
Lewis, C. S. 83
liminal: as place 126
Long, Richard 115, 117–124; *Circle in Africa. Mulanje Mountain Malawi* 119; *Full Moon Circle* 122–124; *A Line Made by Walking* 118; *Tame Buzzard Line* 121; *White Water Falls* 120; *White Water Line* 117, 118

Maasai 47–50
Maclaghan, D. 125
Manet, Edouard: *Le Dejeuner sur l'herbe* 18; *Olympia* 18
manyatta 49, 50
Mappelthorpe, Robert 112
Matisse, Henri 10, 22–30, 86, 99; *Chapel of the Rosary* 23; *Red Studio* 24–28, 30, 102, 126; *Woman Reading* 23
memory 97, 101, 108; visual 10
Miller, J. 28, 63, 107
Milner, M. 24, 76, 77, 125
miracle 37, 38, 75
mnemonic 72
Monterchi 34
moran 49, 50
mother 110; *see also* Bourgeois, Louise
mystery 91, 95; female 35
myth 85

numinosum 85

paint, colour of: blue 17; green 99; red 24–27, 28, 102; *see also* colour as emotional state
Papua New Guinea 61
Paris Salon 17, 18
Parker, D. 101
Paul, Celia 98
La Paz 51–53
perspective 34, 76, 82
Picasso, Pablo 10, 82, 85, 87; *Vollard Suite* 10
Le Pichon, Y. 84
procreation 62, 63
psyche 43; in Renaissance 72
psychoanalysis 76, 108; *see also* Jungian analyst

Quecha 51, 52

rage 29, 30, 110, 114; female 112; *see also* Bourgeois, Louise
Ravilious, Eric 50
Redon, Odilon 10
Renoir, Pierre-Auguste 10, 13–21, 126; *At the Concert* 20; *At the Theatre* 20;

La Loge 6, 19–20; *Les Parapluies* 14–19
repair 110; *see also* Bourgeois, Louise
Rivera, Diego 65–67; *Corrido of the Proletarian Revolution* 65
Rothko, Mark 28, 52
Rousseau, Henri 79–87; *The Hungry Lion* 84; *The Sleeping Gypsy* 80–83, 85, 86; *The Snake Charmer* 79, 80, 84; *Tiger in a Tropical Storm (surprised!)* 6

Samburu 48, 49
San Marco 72, 73
Sansepolcro 32
self 69, 70; multiple 67–70
self-portrait 66–68
Sidoli, M. 43
Solnit, R. 119
space 77; as container 26
Spencer, Stanley 65
splitting 69; *see also* self
Spurling, H. 29

touch 17, 41, 42
Tucker, M. 51
Turner, J. M. W. 50

unconscious 71, 76, 77, 79, 81, 84, 85, 86, 87, 97; collective 62, 84; *see also* dreams

Van Baburen 90
Van Gogh, Vincent 8; *Bedroom at Arles* 6; *Sunflowers* 8, 12
Vermeer, Johannes 87–95; *Girl Reading a Letter by an Open Window* 91–95; *The Procuress* 89–91; *Woman with a Pearl Necklace* 95
voyeur 90

walking 118, 124; as creative space 119
weaving 110, 115
Wolf, B. 94
Wordsworth, William 119

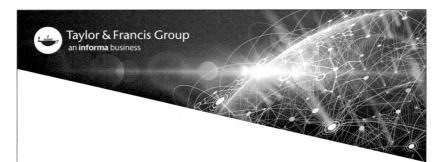